GLADYS PORTUGUES has appeared in *Self* and *Cosmopolitan*, and on the covers of *Ms.*, *American Photographer*, *Muscle and Fitness*, *Shape*, and *Flex* magazines. She has been a guest on the *Phil Donahue* show and appeared in the film *Pumping Iron II*. As a participant in the Women's Olympia international competition, she took the prize for Best Improved Bodybuilder.

JOYCE VEDRAL is a regular contributor to *Muscle and Fitness* magazine, the author of *Now or Never*, the co-author of *Hard Bodies*, and the co-author with Rachel McLish of *Perfect Parts*. Joyce is also an expert on motivational techniques, and has written several books on that subject. She has been a guest on the *Oprah Winfrey* show.

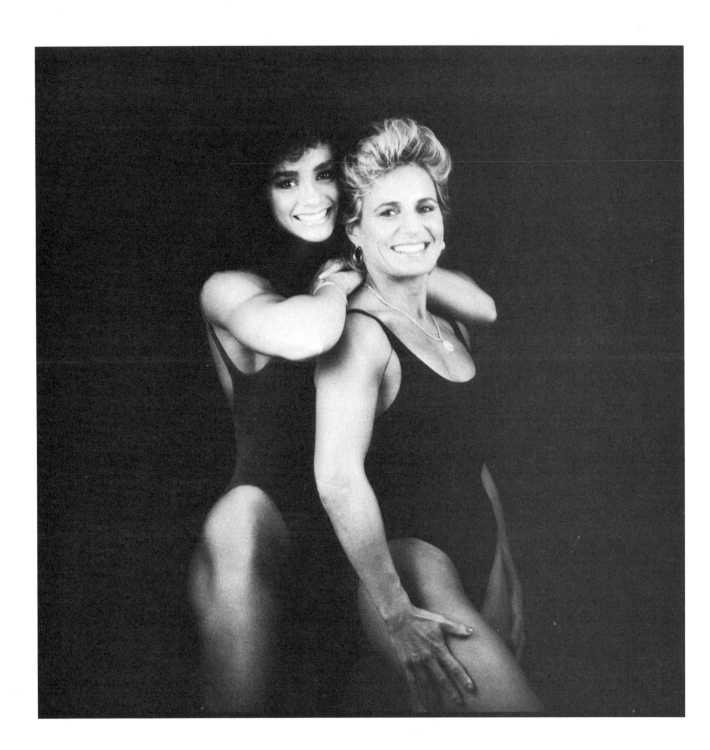

HARD BODIES

Gladys Portugues and Joyce Vedral, Ph.D.

Photographs by Paul B. Goode

A DELL TRADE PAPERBACK

Published by
Dell Publishing
a division of
Bantam Doubleday Dell Publishing Group, Inc.
1540 Broadway
New York, New York 10036

Designed by Richard Oriolo

The trademark Dell® is registered in the U.S. Patent and Trademark Office.

Portugues, Gladys.
Hard bodies.

Bibliography: p.
Includes index.
1. Bodybuilding for women.   2. Exercise for women.
I. Vedral, Joyce L.   II. Title
GV546.6.W64P67   1986   646.7'5
ISBN 0-440-53424-0
Library of Congress Catalog Card Number: 85-16846

February 1986
20   19   18   17   16   15
CWO

This book is dedicated to the women
who believe that by effort they can make changes,
to those who will resculpt their bodies into
the most perfect form possible.

ACKNOWLEDGMENTS

Thank you, Joe Weider, for inventing the scientific principles of bodybuilding upon which this book is based, and for personally helping us to perfect our own physiques.

Thank you, Brian Moss, of Better Bodies Gym and Model Management, for your guidance and vigilance.

Thank you, Mike Alalof, for showing us where to work out.

Thank you, Ken Wheeler, Mohammed Makkawy, and Steve Michalik, for the fine training assistance you have offered.

Thank you, Paul B. Goode, for your artistic photography.

Thank you, professional male and female bodybuilders, for your fine example.

Thank you, Bill Reynolds, for all the fine professional bodybuilding books you have both written and edited.

Thank you, families and friends, for your encouragement, enthusiasm, and support.

Thank you, Nike, for supplying the shoes and workout clothing.

Most important, thank you, Gary Luke, for your astute guidance. Your relentless effort has made all the difference.

CONTENTS

HARD BODIES

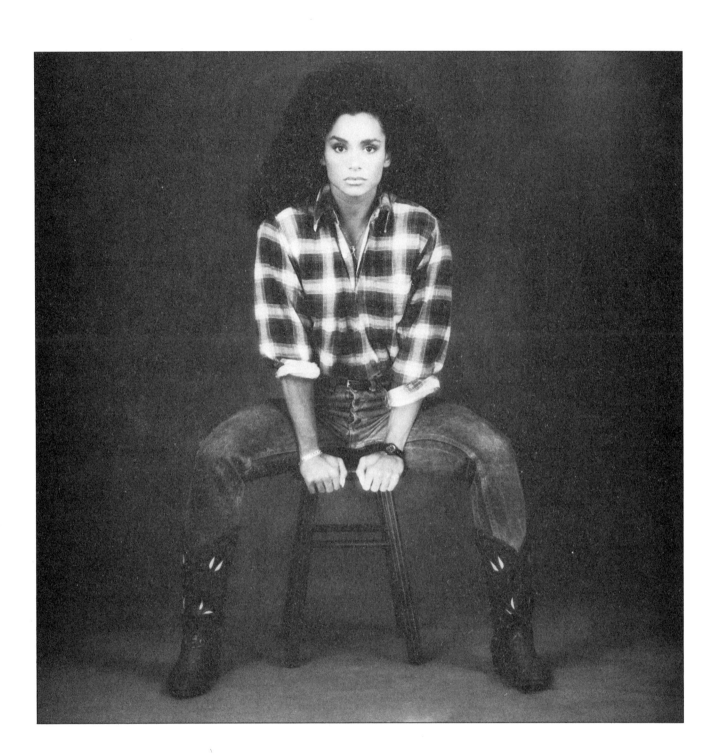

A HARD BODY
IS A SEXY BODY

Women have been frustrated in their efforts to reshape their bodies because they have not consulted the right specialist. If one has an eye problem, one goes to an ophthalmologist; a foot problem, to a podiatrist; a skin problem, to a dermatologist. Take your problem to the wrong specialist and you will not receive the help you need. That's common sense. Yet women seeking to shape their bodies into the most perfect possible form are repeatedly disappointed when they don't get the results they want—after having gone to the wrong specialist.

We have wandered into aerobics classes, where we get heart and lung stimulation. We have tried tennis, where we perfect our game and strengthen arms and legs somewhat. We have joined calisthenics classes, where we are able to reduce some unsightly fat. We have tried everything from running, walking, bike riding, squash, and handball to sailing, horseback riding, and even the martial arts, and still have not achieved the goal: a perfectly shaped, sensual body.

There are many wonderful sports and all kinds of physical activities which benefit us both physically and mentally. The martial arts are great for self-defense and strength training; jogging and running are excellent for burning calories and getting the heart and lungs in shape. Each sport or exercise has its particular specialty and holds its own promise. Which of these activities, however, promises to deliver a perfectly shaped, hard, sexy body? Which of them promises any troublesome body part "rebuilt" until it is in the most attractive possible form? None of them.

Only working out with weights makes that promise. No other activity resculpts sagging muscles and develops the antigravity muscles that keep women looking and feeling young.

We propose a workout program that will not make you into a competitive bodybuilder but will instead utilize the time-tested principles used by bodybuilders to help you sculpt your body into its most perfect form. We have done this for ourselves first, and we have helped hundreds of other women do the same.

Fitness has come to mean firmness, even sensual hardness. Many years ago women were considered desirable only if they were soft and curvaceous. That was also considered feminine and sexy. The problem was, even then, that soft curves were attractive only when the women were in their teens and twenties and still possessed the natural elasticity of youth. But the soft, appealing curves soon developed into loose skin and bunched-up fat (cellulite), and the women's posture indicated loss of vitality. Youth was ended at thirty.

Things have changed. Today women remain young well into their forties and even longer. Fortunately for all of us, soft and loose are out of vogue. Hard and tight is the sensuality of the eighties.

In order to insure the hard body, the shapely muscles, the sleek lines, the planned curves, it is necessary to train carefully with weights. We will help you, first, to evaluate your present body condition; second, to understand exactly what your particular workout routine will involve; third, to learn how to use weights and machines to resculpt your body; and fourth, to fine-tune your routine to meet your particular goals and attack your body problems.

Yes. Weights. But do not worry, we are not planning to turn you into a professional bodybuilder. There are hundreds of books about female bodybuilding. That is the furthest thing from our minds. Nor do we want to see you take on the physical appearance of Charles Atlas. In fact, it would be quite difficult to do that without deliberately tampering with your natural testosterone hormone balance.

Men naturally produce ten times more testosterone than women. That is the hormone that gives men deeper voices, heavier facial hair, and larger muscles and bones than women. Some women take artificial testosterone (steroids) to trick nature and grow bigger muscles than they would develop naturally by lifting weights. The side effects are seen in the lowered voice, the increased facial hair, and finally in the oversized muscles. Such women do in fact resemble men.

Other women, those you may have seen competing in bodybuilding shows, work out in the gym for many more hours than you ever will when following the Hard Bodies program. They train twice a day, often for three hours at a time and six days a week. In addition they use intensified training techniques which we do not recommend.

There is a world of difference between professional competition bodybuilders and you. Your goal is to develop the most sensual, perfectly shaped, hard body possible: one hundred percent femininity and perfect proportion.

Women who train with us are models, actresses, executives—all women who wish to become their most beautiful selves. By using the time-tested principles of Joe Weider, the father of modern bodybuilding, we teach you how to control the gradual reshaping of every part of your body.

You will not be asked to spend many hours in the gym. Four days a week, an hour and a half each time will do it.

We ask you to train each body part in isolation. You will train your chest muscles (pectorals), shoulder muscles (deltoids), and back muscles (latissimi dorsi). Our goal is to give you a firm, uplifted chest, separated breasts, shapely shoulders, and a V-shaped back.

We teach you to train your abdominal muscles, so that your stomach will never again worry you about fat, bulges, or bloat. Before long you'll have tiny, shapely muscles all over your abdominal area. These muscles serve as a girdle to help you naturally keep your stomach tight.

We give you routines for working your biceps to form pretty, sexy arms. We teach you to work on your triceps, located under your biceps, between the armpit and the elbow—an area that soon begins to "hang" on women who don't work out. We teach you to work on your thighs, to reduce or increase them in size—whichever is needed—and to place shapely muscles on them. We help you to tighten your buttocks, to resculpt your hips, and to develop your calves.

By the time we finish with you, you are a new body, a hard body. And you are a strong body.

Many women think that they do not care about strength or hardness, just weight loss. These women are missing the point. What good is a lightweight flabby body?

Weight loss is not really your goal. Fat loss is. And muscle gain. As you lose fat (that thin layer of soft material just under your skin) you will be building your muscles (those shapely formations that give your body curves). The scales may show no change at first because muscles, inch for inch, weigh more than fat. Fat takes up a lot of space, but its spongy composition makes it light. Muscle takes up little space, but its condensed form makes it heavier. Think of a pillow. It takes up more space than a dictionary, yet it weighs much less. For this reason, bodybuilders don't watch the scale, they watch the mirror. Soon your concerns will be "How do I look?" "How do I feel?" Of course, those who are extremely overweight from fat will lose weight eventually, because they will lose more weight in fat than they will gain in muscle.

The goal is to end up with a hard body. But we all start out in different conditions. That's why there are three different workout routines. We make these distinctions: in-between bodies (neither overweight nor underweight), slim bodies (ten pounds or more underweight), and bulky bodies (ten pounds or more overweight). We have provided charts (pp. 55 and 56) for self-evaluation. While weight does not count later, it does in the beginning, when your weight is mostly fat. Later as you become more muscular, the evaluation charts will have less relevance.

If you fall into the slim body category you will train with heavier weights and perform fewer repetitions. The bulky body routine uses light weights and more repetitions. If you are an in-between body, you will gradually change from light weights and high repetitions to heavier weights with low repetitions. Your routine will be tailor-made for *you.*

In two months time you will be taught how to attack troublesome body parts, such as a bulging stomach, large buttocks, skinny legs, hanging triceps, or lumpy hips. You will be shown how to "bomb" the unsightly areas until they meet your standard of perfection. Everything is clearly spelled out in simple steps.

A routine consists of exercises for each body part. For example, a day's routine might consist of three exercises (about twenty minutes) for the chest, three exercises for the shoulders, three exercises for the back, and four exercises for the stomach.

Many women complain that nothing has worked, that losing those bulges and changing those unsightly body parts is impossible. Our clients have a different tale to tell. A thirty-three-year-old woman reshaped her body so completely that after ten months she looked younger than she had looked when she was twenty-five. She brought in a picture to prove it. She was not overweight at twenty-five, nor was she overweight now. It was the reshaping of her body that made all the difference.

Bodybuilding has no age limits. Some of the women who come into the gym are teenagers and some are in their fifties and sixties. Bodybuilding restores vitality. It is the only real weapon one can use to drastically slow and even reverse the signs of aging.

Working out with weights helps to develop and maintain the antigravity muscles. Those are the muscles that control your posture—the way you stand and walk. It is the antigravity muscles that allow us to stand upright and keep us from bowing over in a hunchback position. These are the muscles that keep our shoulders from drooping and our necks from bending downward. They keep our stomachs from protruding. In essence, these are the muscles that keep us from shrinking up and looking old and withered. What is aging, after all, but atrophy, loss of muscle, loss of strength, loss of good posture, loss of elasticity, and loss of vitality and movement.

THE TRAINING EFFECT

The training effect is the carryover of increased physical and mental capacity as a result of disciplined working out in a particular sport or activity.

With the Hard Bodies workout the training effect shows up in many places. It works in the gym in two stages: alarm and then resistance. In the alarm stage, the body is "alarmed" as it is asked to do some new lifting task. In the resistance state, the body marshals its forces, prepares for action, and then acts to conquer the lifting task at hand.

This learned alarm-resistance pattern teaches the individual that growth and change are realities when effort is exerted. The training individual places this information in her subconscious mind, noting that if a demand is made, a response to overcome that demand, even if it is most difficult, can be accomplished. The setting up of this demand-response pattern is the reason that so many women tell us that since they have begun to follow our program, many other areas of their lives have come together in a positive way. It is not unusual for us to hear stories about side-effect success in careers as well as personal relationships.

Lisa, a salesclerk of twenty-six, had been working in a department store for about a year when she began to follow our program. She had studied merchandising in a local college but couldn't find a job as a buyer. After working out for five months she asked for and got a promotion, which was the step before becoming assistant buyer in her department. She says: "Since I've been training I have more self-confidence. I think I can overcome new things. I feel in control. I'm more daring."

Lisa's initial "alarm" at having to take on new responsibilities was combated by "resistance": she marshaled her forces, asked for the promotion, got it, and then overcame all obstacles involved in the new job responsibilities. The "training effect" had carried over into her job situation.

Another young lady who trains with us, Joanne, a thirty-year-old, began working out while in the process of completing a long and difficult divorce. She was at first reluctant to join the gym, fearing that she would not be able to keep her mind on anything, much less learning new workout routines. We explained that since working out requires one's full attention, it actually has a therapeutic effect. The individual is forced to shelve all problems for the time she spends in the gym, and the time off serves as a refreshing release. Often the problem does not seem as drastic when one returns to it. She agreed to give it a try, and we watched her come and go for the next eight months without comment.

Then one day she stopped by to tell us: "It's over. My divorce is settled and everyone is happier than we expected. I even managed to control my temper, and I think that made all the difference. Somehow I think working out helped me with that. For some strange reason I was able to stop myself from flying off the handle. My new calm made it easier to negotiate a settlement. I relate it to what I learned at the gym when I used to find myself ready to give up during my last set. I would think, *No, you have to finish your set,* and I used all the energy I had left to do it. Maybe that self-discipline is what did it for me. Maybe I learned to be that way in life too."

Joanne had learned to apply the training effect to her emotional life. The alarm stage quickly gave way to resistance, and instead of flying off the handle Joanne marshaled her forces, bided her time, and made her point. End result: a satisfactory settlement.

Women who have trained with us tell us they get along better with their boyfriends, are calmer with their children, and are less fearful about trying new things. We suspect that this has something to do with the training effect.

An obvious carryover of the training effect is increased strength. Women who couldn't carry a heavy bag of groceries now have no trouble, and a teacher reported that she no longer waits for the elevator when carrying a carton of paperbacks. "Why waste time," she says. "I just walk up the stairs with them. No problem at all." Those who play tennis or racquetball tell us that they are physically stronger and that their hitting hand is more powerful. Dancers now have more stamina, and models report that they are able to endure much longer shoots with less fatigue.

THE ADDICTION

Small wonder that women become rather upset if they are forced by some uncontrollable life situation to miss a planned workout. What is this strangely addictive quality of working out? Why do women come back to the gym again and again, sacrificing their valuable time and energy, time that could be spent sipping cocktails, watching television, reading a book, or doing anything else? What is it that lures them back even when they are stiff and aching from a previous workout—even after a long workday?

Tara came into our gym an in-between body, but a very soft and weak one. We admired her perseverance as we watched her walk in smiling, four times a week—beginning with the very first week—sometimes looking very stiff and uncomfortable. Two months into her training we asked her how she had felt during her first week. "I was always in pain," she said, "and sometimes I felt as if I could hardly walk."

"Well, why did you keep coming back for more punishment?" we asked.

"Oh," she said, "I felt the pain all right, and the stiffness, but I also felt exhilarated—a sense of a new life. For the first time in my life I was somebody. I had a new feeling of power, and every time I left the gym my mood was so high I thought I could do anything in the world. Now if I miss a workout I feel lazy and loose again. I don't want to feel like those women who are letting their bodies just go to pot. I want to be special, different—and coming here makes me that. I have also become addicted to the admiration I get at work. People are always asking me, 'Going to the gym tonight?' That makes me feel good."

That feeling has been expressed as the runner's high, the dancer's ecstasy, or the spiritual experience. In bodybuilding it is the rush of blood to the muscle, the pump, making the muscle bulge and feel hot. It's the circulation sped up by the repeated lifting and lowering of the weights. It's the transformation of a cold, lethargic body into a hot, working body. It's the beads of sweat on shining skin, the soaked headband as you undress in the locker room, the smell of hard bodies doing hard work. It's the clang of weights and the groan of one more "rep." It's the surge of energy that lasts two and even three hours after the workout, and the clean feeling after a hot shower. The addiction. It sets in. Before you know it, you're hooked.

Not everyone gets hooked right away. Roseanne would shuffle into the gym and reluctantly change into her gym attire, then go through her entire routine in seeming distress, often asking how long before she would be able to stop working out (missing the point that we tried continually to stress to her, that working out must become a lifetime habit). Five months later, Roseanne is a new person. Don't get in her way when she sprints into the gym. She goes directly to the lockers, then quickly reappears and attacks the weights. Her face shows that she means business. With sparkling eyes and pent-up energy, she gets through her workout (doing everything according to strict form) in record time.

No matter how long it takes to become addicted (three weeks is an average), working out soon becomes a part of your life, a necessary habit. Like brushing the teeth or taking a shower, like getting dressed in the morning and putting on makeup; before you know it, working out is no longer up for negotiation. It is a must. Work to be done.

The pump. The high. Feeling like Superwoman. That's what keeps us coming back again and again and again. Food for the stomach, weight-training for the body. One becomes as necessary as the other for physical and mental well-being.

HARD IS SEXY

Hard is beautiful. Hard is sexy. What are the options? Starvation diets which result in soft, slim bodies that are not sensual without clothing? Participation in hit-and-miss sports and activities not designed to totally resculpt the body and to build sensual muscles? Programs that produce a muscle here, a thin spot there?

Is hard sexy and beautiful? Look at the pictures in this book and make a decision. The investment of time now in an intelligent bodysculpting program will last a lifetime.

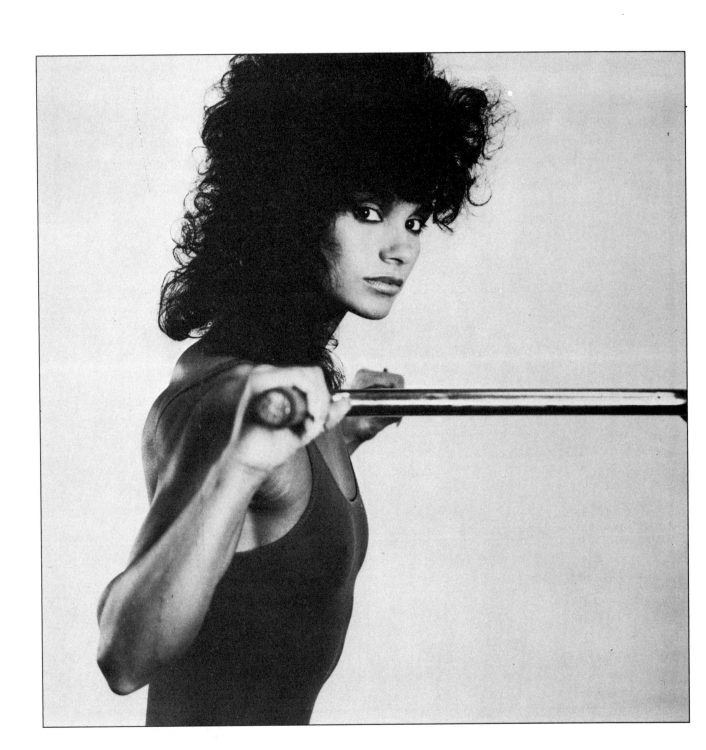

TWO

DOING IT

If you are starting out with a soft body, one that is perhaps oversized around the stomach area, less than ideally formed around the thighs, and maybe a little too large around the hip-buttocks area, it will take an effort to get that hard body.

After a week you may feel tighter and stronger, but no visible results are apparent. In two weeks there will be a "pump," making the muscles seem larger, but the pump will last only a few hours after the workout, when the muscles will return to normal size. In three weeks you will see some muscular development and some reduction of body fat. (An extremely overweight person, however, will have to wait longer to see the muscles—about a month or two. The muscles are growing, but they are hidden under a cushion of fat beneath the skin.)

In a month specific muscles show definite change. The pectorals (chest muscles) become well rounded, the shoulders show definition (pretty lines define the deltoids), and the entire body feels tighter and stronger.

In three months all muscular groups show visible development. A cleavage line is seen in the pectoral area, the deltoids (shoulder muscles) continue to develop shape, the thighs begin to tighten up and show a trace of definition (a line

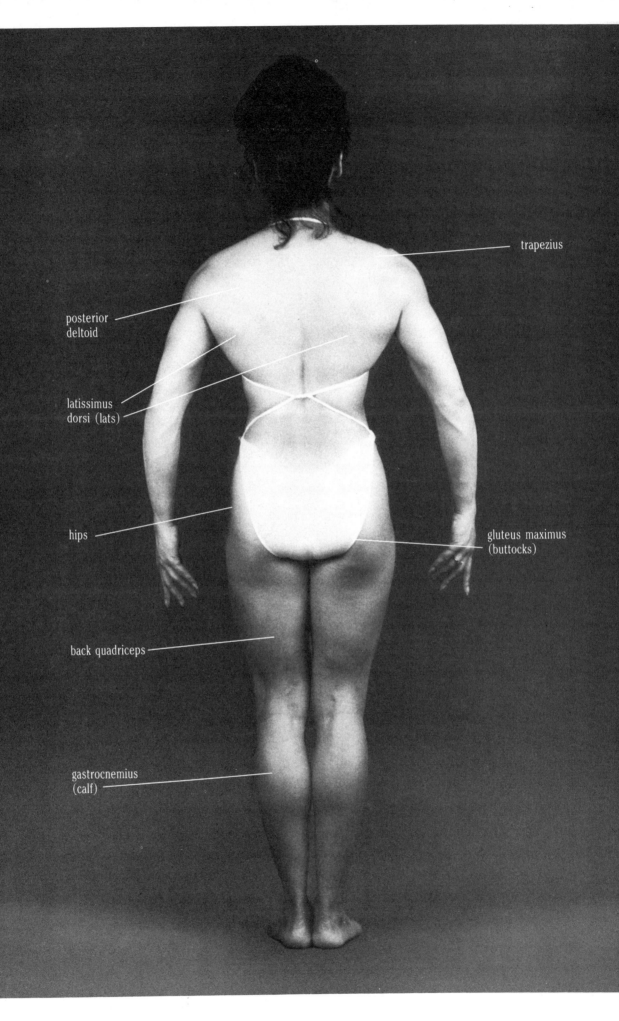

trapezius

posterior
deltoid

latissimus
dorsi (lats)

hips

gluteus maximus
(buttocks)

back quadriceps

gastrocnemius
(calf)

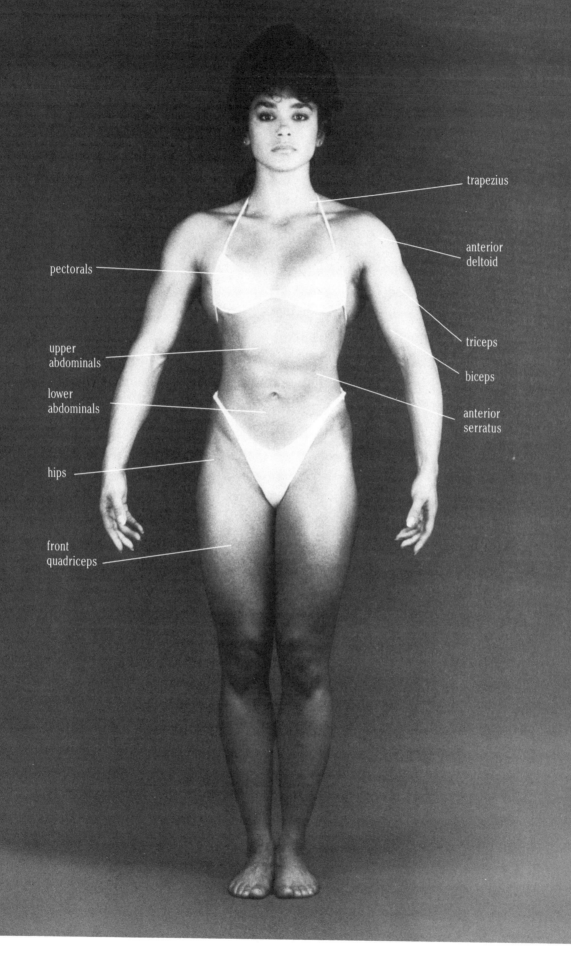

trapezius

anterior
deltoid

pectorals

triceps

biceps

upper
abdominals

lower
abdominals

anterior
serratus

hips

front
quadriceps

separating the thigh muscle can be traced), and the calves begin to develop. The "lats" (side back muscles) do not show growth yet—they take a bit longer— but other small muscles can be seen in your back. The most noticeable growth is in your arms. Your biceps are larger than before, and you can actually "make a muscle." Your triceps (located under your biceps) have begun to tighten slightly.

In six months friends will begin to notice the change, and you will begin to walk with an athletic stride—head held high, arms not hanging down but swinging from strong shoulders, and hips swaying tightly over muscular, well-developed thighs and trim shapely buttocks. By now the lats have begun to widen, giving you the broad-shouldered, narrow-waisted V of an athlete as opposed to the pear-shaped look of a sedentary woman.

In a year the perfectly symmetrical body will be yours, except for a minor area which you are still "bombing" for special results. All excess body fat will be gone and even your triceps will be tight. Each body part will be clearly defined. People will see your biceps, triceps, chest, shoulders, back, thighs, calves, and abdominals.

BODY PARTS

The Hard Bodies workout is muscle-specific. That means we have exercises designed to work on specific muscles. You need to know some basics about your body. Each muscular group is called a body part, and there are seven of them. Take a look at the pictures of Gladys's anatomy as you read our definitions.

BICEPS

The muscle that bulges in the upper arm between the shoulder and the crook of the bent arm is called a biceps. It is the favorite muscle for showing off when someone says "Let me see your muscles."

TRICEPS

The muscle between the elbow and the armpit, on the opposite side of the arm from the biceps, is called a triceps. It is the part that "hangs" on many older or out-of-shape women.

LEGS

Two areas are included in the legs, calves and thighs. The calf is the lower back part of the leg; calves are naturally well-developed on women who wear high-heeled shoes every day or who run a great deal. The thigh is the part of the leg between the knee and the hip; the thigh muscles are the front quadriceps and the back quadriceps. There are exercises for each part of the leg.

CHEST

The chest is located in the breast area, and the muscles under the breasts are called pectorals. We give exercises for lower, upper, and all-over pectoral development.

SHOULDERS

There are two muscles to be developed in each shoulder—the deltoid and the trapezius. The deltoid is located on the front and back shoulder, and the trapezius is located between the neck and the shoulder.

BACK

The back muscles include the "lats" (latissimi dorsi), the teres major, and lots of little muscles all over the back. The smaller muscles of the back are developed first, then the trapezius muscles and the lats. The trapezius is considered both a shoulder muscle and a back muscle.

ABDOMINALS

The abdominal muscles are located between the breast and the upper thigh. They include upper abdominals (above the waist line) and lower abdominals (below the waistline). The abdominal area also includes the serratus muscles located on the side, but the front half of the side. Exercises are given for upper, lower, and serratus muscles of the abdominal area.

TOTAL BODY SCULPTING

In a year's time the entire body will have well-defined muscles and will approach perfection and symmetry. This will have been achieved through the precision of the Hard Bodies workout. Perform exercises in the exact order and in the exact quantity and in the precise manner instructed, and you will rebuild or resculpt your soft body into a hard body. In effect, you will reshape it.

We suggest that you take a before-and-after picture. Take a picture of yourself in a bikini now, and a new one a year later. Your new, finely shaped, symmetrical body will be evident. No matter how good you think you look now, there will be a world of difference in the after picture.

You become an "eye expert." You learn to look at yourself and say "I need more lats." Or "My thighs are too big for my upper body." Such is the power of a seasoned Hard Bodies graduate that she can literally reshape her body according to her desired look. It is only a matter of time and careful workouts. An overall feeling of calm confidence is the end result as you realize that you have the means to make the change you desire, and what keeps you from it is the time and the doing of it. The fear of getting fat is gone forever, and the feeling of being in control of what happens to your body's shape becomes a sure foundation.

WHAT WEIGHT DEMAND DOES TO MUSCLE

In order to realize the goal of a perfectly symmetrical body, it is necessary to cause the muscles to grow at a controlled rate. How, then, does the muscle actually grow? In order to cope with the heavier loads being demanded of them, muscles grow. Muscles are made up of protein—strands of actin and myosin. As muscles are stressed by being asked to push or pull a weight, the muscle tissue is stimulated and blood is pumped into the muscle as it moves in a contracting and expanding motion. Regular and systematic stimulation of the muscle in this fashion is what causes growth. As a greater demand is gradually made upon the muscle by introduction of heavier weight, the muscle works harder (pumps more blood) and is forced to grow larger. This is the foundation of the Hard Bodies workout: the gradual increase of the demand upon specific, isolated muscles. The muscles can do nothing but literally rise to the occasion.

Gradual is important to remember. If, for example, one tried to make a weight leap from a ten-pound dumbbell curl to a fifty-pound dumbbell curl, not only would the muscle refuse to perform the task, but an injury might take place because of the sudden demand. We start you out with a very light weight on each exercise and periodically increase it by a small amount as each weight becomes too easy for you. Each increase is enough to challenge the muscle without stressing it.

If you start out doing a ten-pound dumbbell curl, in about two weeks you might go up to a twelve-pound dumbbell curl, and in another three weeks you may be strong enough to go up to a fifteen-pound dumbbell curl. You will never advance to a higher weight unless you feel that the lighter weight is no longer a challenge.

WHAT A WORKOUT ENTAILS

On one training day you will work chest, shoulders, back, and abdominals, on another training day you will work biceps, triceps, legs, and abdominals.

On the day you work chest, shoulders, back, and abdominals, here is what you will be doing.

You will work your chest first. Your first chest exercise will be the bench press, and you will use a bench press machine. The next chest exercise will be the cable crossover, using one of the machines in the gym. The third and final chest exercise will be an incline flye, using a dumbbell.

Each of the chest exercises may require different beginning weights. For example, on the bench press you may be pushing a bar weighing forty pounds, while on the cross bench pullover you may be lowering a dumbbell weighing fifteen pounds. On the cable crossover you may be pulling two eight-pound weights. The starting weight is determined by the nature of the particular exercise. Weight is not the issue. Muscle challenge—"work"—is the issue, as well as the strict performance of the exercise (as stressed in the exercise descriptions).

The entire chest routine should take fifteen to twenty minutes; when you are finished, your chest should feel tight and "pumped" (bigger and rounder from the inflow of blood into that area).

After having completed your chest routine, you will immediately move on to shoulders. You need not rest: the chest will be resting while you work your shoulders. Your first shoulder exercise will be the military press to the front. You will use a barbell of perhaps twenty-five pounds. The second shoulder exercise will be a side lateral raise using perhaps a five-pound dumbbell, and the third shoulder exercise might be an upright row using a twenty-five pound barbell. After doing each of the three exercises for the correct number of repetitions and sets (to be explained later), your shoulders will be tight and pumped. You will be able to rest your shoulders as you keep on exercising, because you will move directly to the back exercises.

The first back exercise will be a seated pulley row using a pulley machine at perhaps a forty-pound weight. Next you will do a dumbbell bent row of about fifteen pounds, and finally lat machine pulldowns to the back using, say, fifty pounds. You will have done three exercises for each body part so far.

Now you may feel like stopping, but since you know there is only one more body part to go, abdominals, you will manage to finish.

You will first do sit-ups on a flat board, then crunches against a bench, then Roman chair sit-ups with a weight (using the Roman chair apparatus), and finally leg raises using a straight board. Notice that abdominals require extra exercises. This is because abdominals are rather stubborn and require more training. Because they are small muscles, they can be trained every day without fatigue, and they are the only muscle group you'll exercise every time you work out.

By the time you finish abdominals, you will experience the mixed feeling of triumph and exhaustion. You will walk with a devil-may-care, almost defiant attitude one minute, and the next, you will be dragging your body wondering if you are going to make it. In all, you will feel victorious and superior.

GRADUAL WEIGHT INCREASE

Each workout will make you a little stronger, and as you get stronger you will gradually increase the weight that you lift. For example, the first two weeks of the bench press might entail the use of forty pounds for the first set. After a couple of weeks forty pounds becomes too light and the first set will begin with fifty pounds. In three weeks time that beginning weight of fifty pounds is too easy, so it is increased to sixty pounds, and so on. Naturally there is a time when one remains at the same beginning weight for a few months or so. The point is, gradual weight increase makes muscles grow.

FOUR TIMES A WEEK

When training for something, you have to do just that: train. This involves the systematic devotion of a block of time to the activity; otherwise the expected results will not be achieved.

In order to turn your soft body into a hard body, it is necessary to devote four days a week, one and a half hours each day. No exceptions. The commitment must be made and kept or we cannot guarantee results. Working out must become a priority in your life.

If a person works out only once a week, all that person achieves is weekly muscle soreness and the burning of about seven hundred calories. No change takes place in the body, because the muscles are not being challenged enough.

Working out only twice a week serves as a tease to the muscles. They are challenged to grow, and just when they are ready to do so, they are left to rest, so they instead remain the same size.

Working out three times a week does achieve some results, but not much. Four times a week is the magic number. The extra day provides the missing link, and the body's muscles respond dramatically.

Working out five days a week is not necessary, although some people like to go to the gym an extra day. No harm is done, but we find that most people experience excellent muscular development with four training days a week.

Training six days a week is fine for some, and those who wish to lose body fat often do this to speed up the process. We would rather see such people do an extra half hour of aerobic exercise on those extra days, because training six days a week can fatigue the body as well as the mind and hinder the progress. Six days a week is for the professional bodybuilders.

No professional bodybuilder would suggest training seven days a week. Perhaps the idea of resting on the seventh day is more than a poetic expression or a religious truth. It seems quite clear that the body needs at least one day of rest a week. People who have tried to train for more than six days in a row have incurred frequent injuries. If you won't give the body a rest, it will demand one on its own by setting you up for an injury.

Time can be "found" in many places. One of them is in the space allowed for television viewing. Most people spend at least ten hours a week watching TV. If you gave up six of those hours (1½ times 4) you would still have four hours to sit in front of the tube.

Relaxing, by the way, is what bodybuilding ultimately is. "After I walk out of the gym," says Jody, a twenty-eight-year-old executive, "all the tension is gone. It's better than therapy, and so much less expensive."

But time is limited, after all, and if you work a nine-to-five day, those gym hours have to be carefully planned ahead of time or you simply will not get them into your busy week. Many women go directly to the gym from work, before having dinner. They manage to get to the gym by 5:30 and begin their workout by 5:45. By 7:15 they are finished, by 7:30 they are out of the gym, and their evening is free. They do this, say, on Monday, Tuesday, Thursday, and Friday, taking Wednesday off for a change of pace. Other women go Monday through Thursday, leaving the weekend free. Still others work out on the weekend days and on two weeknights.

There are as many schedules as there are personalities. But there is one constant: the schedule must be kept. Never let moods direct your action. Once you are in the gym doing your first repetition you will be glad you didn't give in to that urge to skip a workout. Be tough. Work hard for a hard body.

MUSCLE TO FAT

Many women fear that if they work out and achieve muscular development, it will all turn to fat once they stop. Nothing could be further from the truth. What actually happens is that when a person develops muscles through weight training and then stops training, the person's muscles shrink back to a smaller size because not as much work is being demanded of them. But the person will not gain fat unless she eats more calories than she is burning. Many times a woman who stops training becomes bored or depressed and eats more than she did when she was training without realizing it. Also, unless she finds another way to burn up seven hundred calories four times a week, she will of course eventually gain back some of the body fat she lost.

The main thing to remember is, muscle cannot physically be transformed into fat and fat cannot be transformed into muscle: they are entirely different substances.

MUSCLE SORENESS AND PAIN

"No pain no gain" is a familiar expression in the bodybuilding world. Unless the muscle is challenged to the point of discomfort (at least in the beginning) you can be sure that nothing is happening and you are wasting your time.

"After my first workout," says Sarah, a thirty-year-old fashion designer, "I felt like crawling out of the gym on all fours, and the next morning I felt even worse. It was a good soreness, though, and I felt as if I were finally getting to my body where it counts, to muscles I had neglected for years. After about two weeks I didn't feel sore anymore."

The morning after the day you train, your muscles will be sore. The truth is, you will hurt, but it is a very bearable pain.

Muscle soreness occurs because your muscles are not used to being expanded and contracted quite so much: they are not used to being asked to work so hard for so long. The ligaments (which connect your bones to other bones) and the tendons (which connect your muscles to your bones) are really being given a surprise. The Hard Bodies workout starts slowly to minimize the soreness.

SEVERE PAIN AND INJURY

There is a vast difference between normal muscle soreness and the severe pain which accompanies injury. The kind of pain that accompanies injury is sharp and arresting, usually making it impossible to continue working out.

Although a medical exam is advised before starting any new physical fitness program, working out with weights is probably one of the safest fitness programs available. There is very little danger of injury in the gym because you are in control of the weights. In other sports you are at the mercy of the game. Even tennis players get hurt at times in a wild dart for the ball. They often twist an ankle, pull a ligament, or tear knee cartilage. The ball controls their actions. In the Hard Bodies workout, on the other hand, you control the weight.

Several types of injuries can occur when working out with weights. Fascia injuries affect the fibrous membrane that covers and supports the skin and unites it with the underlying tissue. It is the basic packaging tissue of the body. The fascia encloses the muscles, and when it is torn (by a sudden jerk or pull) it becomes inflamed. The muscle may even bulge through the fascia, causing severe pain. When this happens, the area must be wrapped with an Ace bandage and allowed to rest for a few weeks. This does not mean that the individual must stop working out, but she must stop doing those exercises that may aggravate the injury.

Another type of injury is tendinitis, inflammation of the tendon. This occurs when the tendons are severely overstressed. Tennis players often experience tendinitis in the elbow ("tennis elbow"); runners often experience it in the knee joint. Careless bodybuilders can get tendinitis if they do not increase their weight load gradually and if they neglect to control the weight as they lower and raise it (that is, if they become careless about following strict exercise form).

Ligament injuries can occur in the gym (especially in the shoulder or knee joints) if the individual violently lunges with a weight or suddenly jerks a weight. Such injuries will not occur if the rules stressed in this book are followed.

The least dangerous of all injuries are bruises. These come from a direct blow with an object, and in the gym that object is a weight. For example, if one is not concentrating (we emphasize concentration), one can hit oneself in the chin when doing a barbell curl.

Bruises bring discoloration, which is caused by bleeding just beneath the skin. The discoloration goes away in a week to ten days.

When an injury occurs, there is some swelling. The greater the injury, usually, the greater the swelling. The area is packed with extra water produced by cellular waste materials. The injury is actually splinted by the excess water; your body has produced water bags to protect the area from further injury. Yet too much swelling can be very painful; to keep it at a minimim, the injured person should apply ice packs several times a day for the first few days.

GYM VERSUS HOME

Many people wonder why it is necessary to work out in a gym, thinking they could save a lot of travel time by working out at home.

Working out at home brings many problems, and not too many people are highly enough motivated to overcome them. First, there is no camaraderie to inspire you. Then there are distractions such as the telephone, the television, the refrigerator, a good book, or even the bed. Finally, there is the expense of buying the equipment. Dumbbells and barbells are not too expensive, but few people could afford the Nautilus machines, the Universal Gym equipment, or even the free-standing pulley machines that are necessary for a complete workout. While it is true that there are barbell and dumbbell substitutes for many of the machines, we feel that the machines add that finishing touch to the workout. They not only add variety and thus make the workout less boring, but they make it possible to use heavier weights with a greater degree of safety.

Working out in a gym also provides an atmosphere of energy. The electricity of "men and women at work" sparks one to pump harder, and the look of approval or the word of encouragement from another gymgoer can make all the difference.

The gym provides people who are able to offer you tips and training advice, and at the gym you can usually find a ready training partner. It isn't necessary to make plans to work out with someone. There is always someone who will ask "What are you working today?" and is willing to work out with you.

The gym is also a good place to make new friends. After a workout is over it is fun to converse with others who have also pushed themselves through a hard workout and are on the after-workout high.

FINDING A GYM

Choosing the right gym is important. Don't be lured by thick rugs and fancy saunas or steam baths. Most bodybuilding gyms have none of these. What they do have is a locker room and a shower. That's all you really need. A no-frills gym is a less expensive gym.

If the gym owner or manager does not encourage you to work out in muscle groups (three exercises for the chest, for example, three sets each exercise, nine sets in all, then three exercises for the shoulders . . .) but insists that you circuit-train (one exercise for every body part each time you work out), do not join that gym. It is an aerobics-beauty gym, and you will not make progress. It will be impossible to resculpt your body with muscles by doing circuit training. A year later you will see no significant change in your body. Even if the manager tells you that you can work out in your own way, be careful: in a gym that stresses circuit training, you may find it hard to use a machine, to do three consecutive sets because there will be people milling around waiting. If you allow them to interrupt your sets, your routine will be adversely affected, as you will be forced to rest longer than you should. Your whole workout will be one of waiting and apologizing for using the machines.

One sign of a good gym is a serious working atmosphere. If there is a lot of chatting going on on the gym floor, the gym is a socializing gym. If people are standing around waiting for machines, bodybuilding and bodyshaping are not top priority. Serious bodybuilders don't wait around—they move to another machine.

An important factor to consider in joining a gym is the leadership. Does the manager know about the kind of routines we stress in this book? A key question to ask is "Do you encourage working out on a split routine?" You may not understand this question yourself right now, but in any gym that stresses serious bodybuilding and bodysculpting, the staff would know that the purpose of split routines is to give the muscles a chance to rest and grow.

Finally, look around at the equipment. Make sure there are plenty of weights and a variety of machines. Make sure the men are not segregated from the women and that women are not restricted to certain equipment and certain areas. If this is the case, you will not have the equipment you need to execute all the routines prescribed in the Hard Bodies workout. There are plenty of gyms that allow women all the privileges of men. Don't let yourself be restricted. Besides, it's more fun to work out with the men.

No matter which gym you choose, you will not need too much help, because this book will serve as your trainer. All you need do is take this book to the gym with you and follow the training guide for your body form. The only questions you will have to ask the gym manager are questions such as "Where are the ten-pound dumbbells?" and "Which machine can I use to do my lat pulldowns?" You won't have to ask how to use the machine; the pictures and the instructions tell you all you need to know.

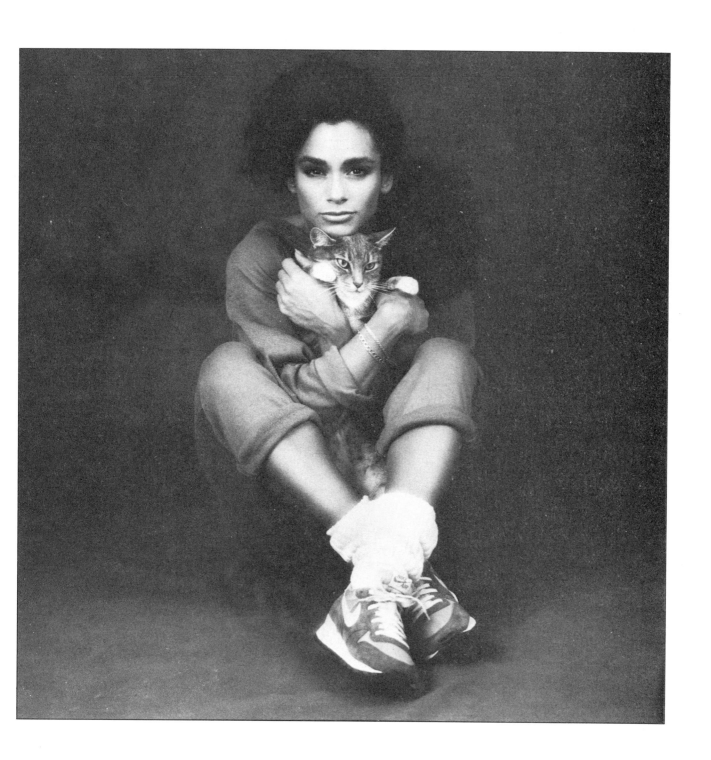

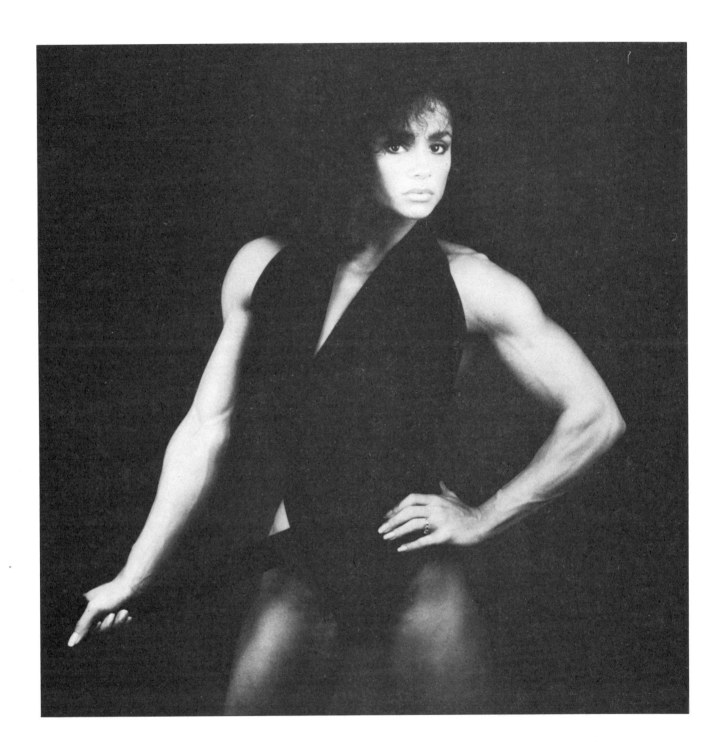

THE BASICS

In order to sculpt your body into its most perfect form, it is necessary to utilize certain principles involving the controlled use of weights. This chapter will provide simple explanations of the basic terms you will need to become familiar with so that you can work out intelligently and get results.

REPETITION (REP)

One full movement of an exercise from start to midpoint and back to the starting point again is called a repetition, or rep. In the bench press, for example, a repetition is the lowering of the bar to the chest and the raising of the bar back up to starting position.

SET

A group of reps is called a set. One performs a series of sets by taking a fifteen- to forty-five-second rest between sets. In the bench press, for example, a set is the lowering and raising of the bar back to starting position fifteen times. There are usually three sets per exercise, so in the bench press one would do fifteen reps, rest, do another fifteen reps, rest, and then do the final set of reps.

EXERCISE

The actual prescribed group of movements being performed—for example, the bench press—is an exercise.

REST

The pause between sets (usually fifteen to forty-five seconds is called a rest). This pause allows the muscle to regain strength for the next set. In the bench press, for example, one would do one set of fifteen repetitions, rest for, say, thirty seconds, do another set of fifteen repetitions, rest for another thirty seconds, perform the final set, and rest another thirty seconds before moving to the next exercise.

ROUTINE

A series of different exercises, each performed a given number of sets, is called a routine. For example, you will do three different exercises consisting of three sets each for your chest, totaling nine sets for your chest. All the sets for a given body part are your routine for that body part. For example, if you do three sets of bench press, three sets of flyes, and three sets of cable crossovers for your chest, those nine sets are called your chest routine.

WORKOUT

The entire bodybuilding session for a given day, consisting of the total sets you do for all body parts that day, is called a workout. For example, on a given day you may be working your chest, your shoulders, your back, and your abdominals. Your entire workout for that day will consist of nine sets for chest, nine sets for shoulders, nine sets for back, and twelve sets for abdominals. There will be thirty-nine total sets in your workout for that day.

FREE WEIGHTS

Barbells and dumbbells are called *free weights* because they can be carried around the gym freely and are not fixed to the ground as are the machines. A *barbell* is a bar to which weights (plates) can be added by attaching them to holding devices (collars). Some barbells have permanently attached weights. A *dumbbell* is a short weight that can be held in one hand and thus can be used to exercise one arm at a time. Both dumbbells and barbell plates have the poundage clearly marked on them.

MACHINES

Most gyms today have a combination of machines. The most familiar brand names are Universal Gym and Nautilus. Universal Gym machines operate on pulleys, and the resistance of the weight being pulled or pushed stays the same all the time. Pulley machines operate the same way. Nautilus machines, on the other hand, operate on cams (curved wheels mounted on rotating shafts). The Nautilus machine, which is a newer invention than the Universal Gym machine, functions to increase weight resistance as more pressure is applied. When a machine is suggested for an exercise, it can usually be done on either a Universal Gym, a Nautilus machine, or another brand-name machine. Machines are valuable because they help to prevent accidents, when working with heavy or awkward weights.

PROGRESSION

Progression is the principle of continually and gradually adding weight to your sets (over a period of weeks or months) so that the muscle is forced to work harder. As a result of being forced to work harder, the muscle grows in size and density, becoming more shapely. For example, for your chest routine, you start out by performing three sets of the bench press. The first week you train, you perform your first set with thirty pounds, your second set with forty pounds, and your third set with fifty pounds. After two weeks your first set is too easy with thirty pounds, so you start out with forty pounds and do your second set with fifty pounds and your final set with sixty pounds. In another three weeks you find that your first set is again too easy, so you increase it to sixty pounds, and so on. (You may not actually progress at this pace, but this illustrates the idea of progression.)

PUMP

The expanded muscle is said to be pumped when it is filled with blood that has been pumped into it because of the vigorous movement of the repetitions of the various exercises. For example, when your chest muscles seem enlarged after your chest routine, people might say, "Your chest is really pumped."

DEFINITION

When the state of a muscle is clearly visible because of absence of excess bodyfat, it is said to be defined. Striations and veins are often visible. For example, when you can see thin lines going outward from the center of your chest, you have achieved definition in your chest area. Definition comes with lots of repetitions as bodyfat is burned away, and is assisted by proper low-fat dieting.

SPLIT ROUTINE

In order to get the most out of working out, it has been discovered that it is best to rest the muscles (except for the abdominals) one day before working them again. The split routine was invented by Joe Weider to ensure that muscles grow to their optimum size without wasted energy and counterproductive effort. If the chest, shoulders, and back are worked on Monday, for example, the biceps, triceps, and legs are worked on Tuesday. (Abdominals are worked every workout day because they require more stress.) If the chest, shoulders, and back are again worked on Wednesday, the biceps, triceps, and legs are again worked on Thursdays. Each body part is worked twice a week (except for abdominals, which are worked four times a week). The split routine allows muscles to rest and recover from the workout. They actually need this rest time in order to grow. Overtraining the muscles by working them every day will result in little visible muscle growth. Instead of growing, they remain the same because they burn themselves out.

Some people wonder why we do not suggest that all the muscles be worked on one day and rested the next. In this way, they argue, it would be possible to work out only two days a week. This would not be a good idea because trying to work all the muscle groups on one day would result in fatigue and improper execution of exercises. The individual would be too tired to concentrate by the time she got to the second half of her workout and would end up with a lopsided muscular development.

SLEEP AND REST

In order to grow, muscles need rest, and muscles rest well while you are sleeping. After a hard workout your body needs time to remove the waste by-products produced by the workout and to refuel the muscles with glycogen and oxygen. If a muscle is not given a full day of rest to recover, it will not have enough time to be refueled and it will not only refuse to grow, it may even shrink. This is why we insist upon the split routine, and why we insist that you get between six and eight hours of sleep, depending upon what your body needs.

Working out without the proper amount of sleep will take a toll on concentration. The temptation to do incomplete repetitions or to rush through the workout will be greater than usual. We do not suggest, however, that you skip a workout just because you did not get enough sleep the night before. It is far better to keep up the discipline of working out, even when tired, than to give in to the tired feeling and stay home. If you work out without enough sleep, eventually your body will direct you to bed at the right time because it will "remind" you of how you will feel the next day when you work out without the right amount of rest. This instinctive method will regulate your sleep-rest patterns, but you must tune in to it and cooperate.

WARM-UPS

Before beginning the workout it is necessary to do some stretching and some aerobics. Walking briskly for five minutes or riding the stationary bike for the same amount of time will take care of the aerobics. Running around the gym for five minutes or jumping rope or doing jumping jacks for the same amount of time would also do the trick. Any activity that gets the heart pumping and the blood circulating is fine, as long as it isn't overdone and doesn't deplete the needed energy for the workout.

Stretches should be kept quite simple and can be done in five minutes. See Chapter Four for a series of stretches that will take you under five minutes.

BASIC AND ISOLATION EXERCISES

Basic exercises work the large muscles of the body and are done with relatively heavy weights. An example of a basic exercise for the chest is the bench press. The weight of the bench press would be at least thirty pounds even for a very weak person. An isolation exercise, on the other hand, works a smaller section of the muscle group and is done with a relatively lighter weight. An example of an isolation exercise for the chest is the incline flye. This exercise is done on an incline bench (a bench slanted upward from the floor) with light weights. A very weak person, for example, would use an eight-pound weight in each hand when doing an incline flye. This would be equivalent to the thirty pounds used on the bench press. The incline flye stresses the upper area of the chest muscles (pectorals), while the bench press stresses the entire area of the chest muscles (pectorals). The Hard Bodies workout provides you with the correct balance of basic and isolation exercise.

PYRAMIDING

Increasing weights with each set of an exercise is known as pyramiding. The traditional method of pyramiding is to increase the weight slightly with each set of an exercise and then gradually decrease it with each set until the original weight is reached, so that a "pyramid" is formed. For example, if one starts out with thirty pounds for the first set of a bench press, then goes to forty pounds for the second set and fifty pounds for the third, then returns to forty pounds for the fourth set and thirty pounds for the fifth and final set, a pyramid has been formed. A modified form of pyramiding is to gradually increase the weight until you reach the pinnacle of the pyramid and stop there. For example, the individual would go from thirty to forty to fifty pounds on the bench press and stop. Another word for modified pyramiding is *stacking*. In this book *pyramiding* is used to refer to modified pyramiding. Full pyramiding is more advanced than is necessary for our workouts. In pyramiding, the reason the weight can be increased is that we allow you to perform fewer reps when the weight is raised. In other words, the weight is raised at the expense of a few repetitions. For example, the individual would do fifteen reps for the first set at thirty pounds, twelve reps for the second set at forty, and ten reps for the third set at fifty. This method provides the opportunity for maximum muscle development and must be used by both slim and in-between bodies. Bulky bodies use the method only if they can still squeeze out the minimum of twelve repetitions for the last set. They are on a special program to burn maximum fat and therefore must never go below twelve repetitions. We are giving them the aerobic effect of working out with the anaerobic effect of working with weights. Pyramiding allows for a natural warm-up (the first set being rather light) and it helps to avoid boredom (sets of unvarying weight and repetitions being rather tedious).

HEAVY VERSUS LIGHT

In order to achieve the specific Hard Bodies goal, it is necessary to utilize the heavy versus light principle. Those who wish to put on maximum mass (very thin people) must use heavy weights and low repetitions. Those who wish to reduce their size (eliminate excess fat) while shaping and developing muscle must use light weights and high repetitions. Those who are neither thin nor bulky will use a combination of heavy weights and light weights. Heavy weights and low reps build mass; light weights and high reps reduce size and give shape. A person with skinny thighs doing squats would do ten repetitions of seventy pounds for the first set, eight repetitions of eighty pounds for the second set, and six repetitions of ninety pounds for the third set. As soon as the first set became easy enough to get more than ten repetitions, she would start with eighty pounds, and so on. If, on the other hand, a person had big thighs and wanted to reduce them, she would do the first set of squats with fifty pounds and do fifteen repetitions. She would do the second set with sixty pounds only if she could get at least twelve repetitions, preferably fifteen. Her third set would consist of the minimum of twelve repetitions at whatever weight she could handle.

TRAINING PARTNERS

Many people prefer working out with a friend who plays the role of a training partner. The training partner can be useful in preventing injury and can also aid one psychologically by giving encouragement. Some people, however, prefer to work alone, claiming that a training partner is a drain of energy and that a partner slows them down. The method of working with a partner demands that the partner "spots" (watches) you while you do a set, after which you rest and spot the partner while he or she does a set. Sometimes the partner's set may take longer than your normal set, and you are slowed down. It isn't necessary to have a training partner, because if a spotter is needed it is a simple matter of signaling anyone who is nearby in the gym. This person could assist you for that particular set, and then you would be free to continue the workout at your own pace.

VISUALIZATION AND CONCENTRATION

Perhaps the most important principle of working out with weights is that of visualization and concentration; without the mind, the body would do nothing. The mind must be used to *visualize* the way the desired body will look when it is completely resculpted. Imagine your hard body. It is necessary to stand in front of the mirror and picture the ideal body you wish to have. Do this at least twice a week, in a bikini or without clothing, imagining the excess body fat melting away and being replaced with shapely muscles. With this mental image of yourself, your body will gradually form itself into that image. This works because such visualization helps the subconscious brain form a "plan" that will realize itself in time. (The area that handles such planning is the right hemisphere of the brain.)

   Another important employment of the mind comes into play in the gym when you are working out. Each time a repetition is performed, the mind must be employed to concentrate on that particular muscle and that muscle only. When working the biceps with a barbell, for example, it is necessary to picture the biceps contracting and growing larger as the barbell is raised, and to see the biceps stretching and filling with oxygen as the barbell is lowered. As the exercise is performed, the mental image of the muscle growing must be kept in the mind at all times. In effect, you must actually tell your muscle to grow as you exercise it. Progress can be increased by more than fifty percent through concentration and visualization, and this principle is utilized by champion bodybuilders as well as actresses, models, and competitors in all major sports. Visualization and concentration cannot be emphasized enough, and for this reason you will notice that it is continually mentioned throughout the book.

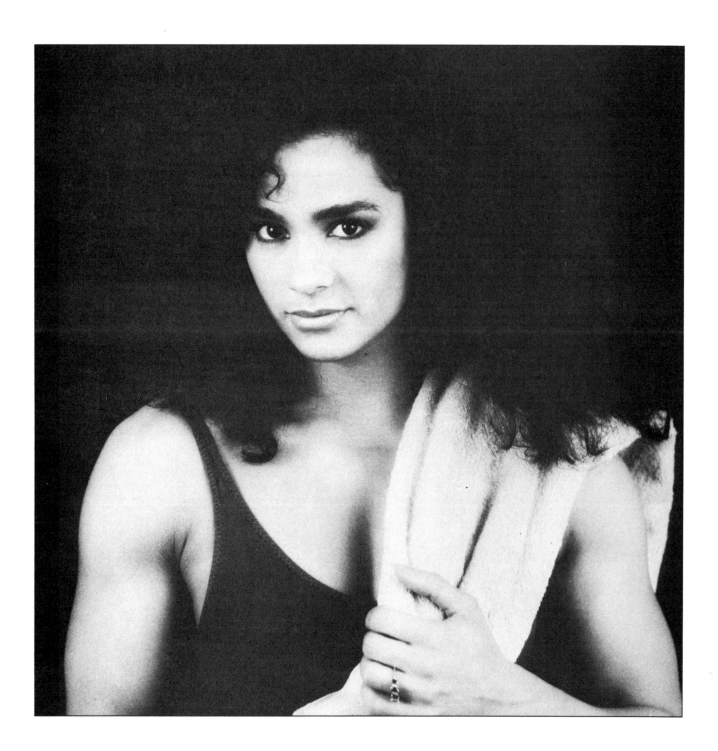

THE FIVE-MINUTE
WARM-UP

Stretches are important. The exercises provided in this chapter are designed to warm up the major and minor muscle groups, and to prepare the body for the workout. These exercises can be performed in five minutes.

BICYCLE

This stretch loosens the entire body and especially stretches the hip area.

DIRECTIONS

- Lie on the floor and raise your legs straight up.

- Place your hands on your hips and raise your hips until your weight is supported by your shoulders. Hold your hips up with your hands. Your elbows are resting on the floor for support.

MOVEMENT

- Move your legs in a bicyclelike motion. (Be sure to move in a full circular motion, bringing your knees as close to your body as possible.)

- Do this for 45 seconds and stop.

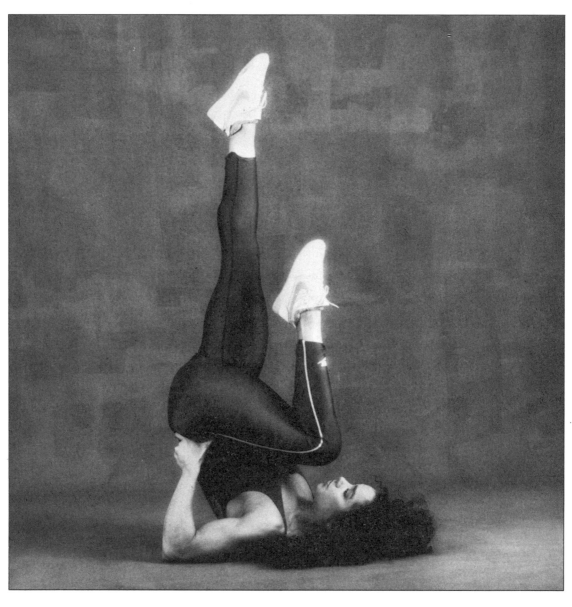

BICYCLE

REACHING

This stretch loosens the shoulder area as well as the biceps, triceps, and forearms.

DIRECTIONS	• Stand up with your feet shoulder width apart and raise both arms directly above your head.

MOVEMENT	• Try to reach the ceiling with one arm at a time, raising your heel with the reaching arm. • Continue this movement, alternating one arm and then the other arm. Do this five times for each arm.

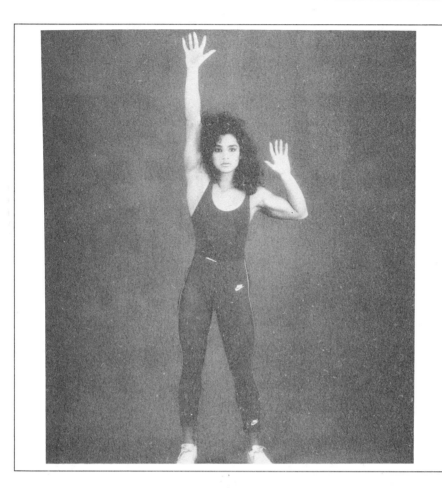

REACHING (START)

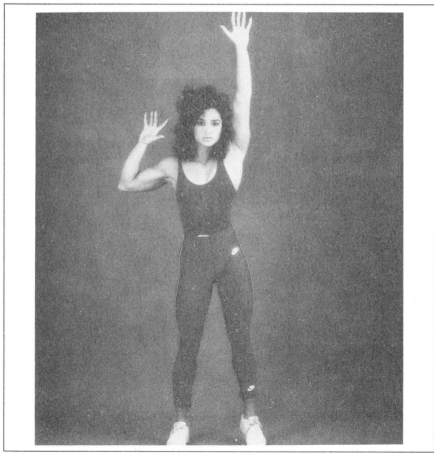

REACHING (FINISH)

BACK BEND

This stretch lengthens the back muscles and loosens the shoulders, abdominals, and front thighs.

DIRECTIONS

- Stand straight up with legs shoulder width apart.

MOVEMENT

- Lean backwards until your hands are touching and holding your thigh just above the knee bend area.

- Remain in that position for 10 seconds and rest for 5 seconds.

- Repeat the movement once.

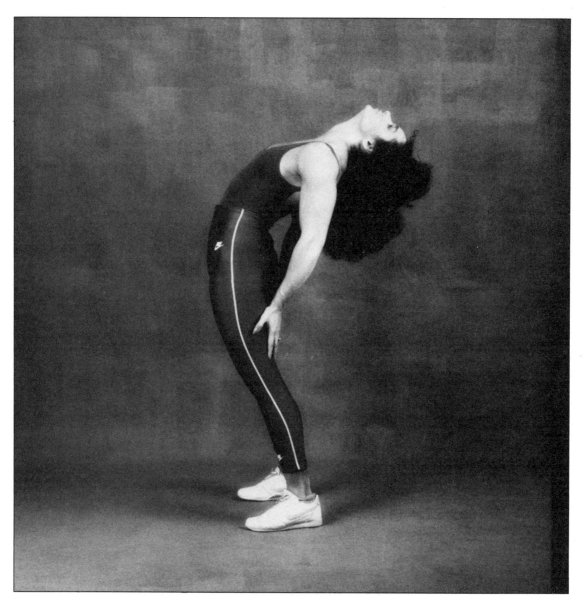

BACK BEND

THIGH STRETCH

This exercise stretches your thigh as well as your front lower leg and ankle.

DIRECTIONS

- Stand with feet shoulder width apart.

- Grasp your right ankle with your right hand.

MOVEMENT

- Slowly pull your ankle toward your waist until you have pulled it as high as you can.

- Hold in that position for 7 seconds and repeat the movement for the other leg.

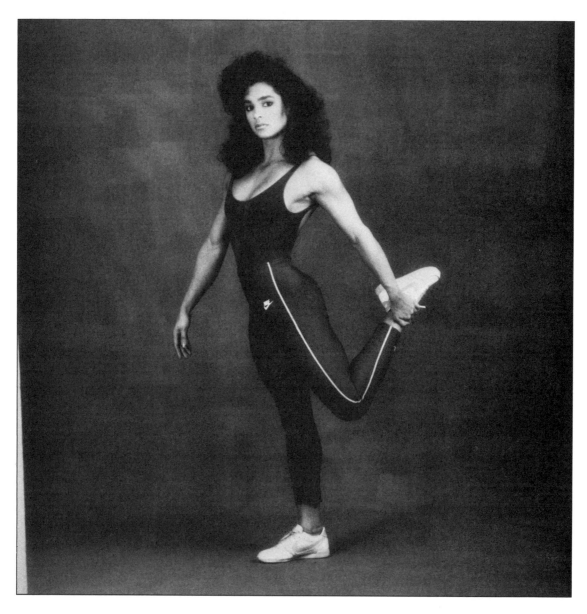

THIGH STRETCH

TOTAL BODY HANG

This stretch emphasizes the back and neck areas but provides a stretch for the entire body.

DIRECTIONS

- Stand with your legs shoulder width apart.

MOVEMENT

- Slowly bend at the waist until your upper body is parallel with the floor.

- Loosen your body and let your arms hang limply down as if they were about to fall onto the floor.

- Remain in this position for about 15 seconds.

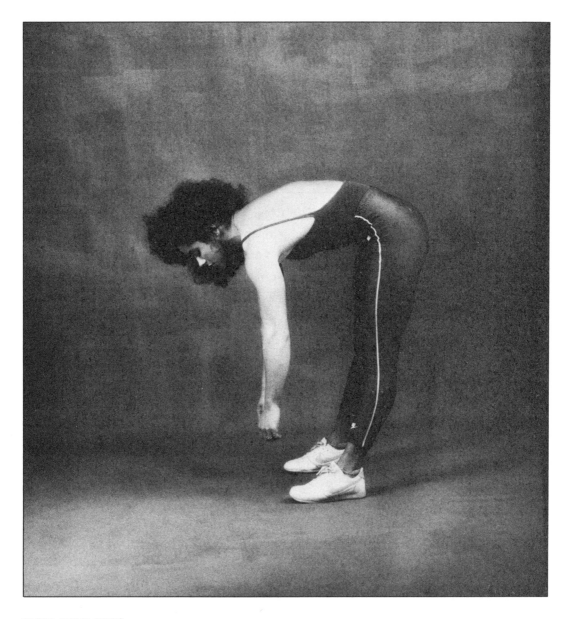

TOTAL BODY HANG

SIDE STRETCH

This stretch loosens the waist and upper side body area.

DIRECTIONS	• Stand with feet shoulder width apart and raise your left arm above your head in an arclike position.
MOVEMENT	• Slowly lean toward your right side, bending at the waist and letting your right arm graze your right knee as your left arm arcs over your head, pulling your body into the stretch. Remain in this position for 5 seconds. Keep your hips straight ahead. • Repeat this movement for the right side.

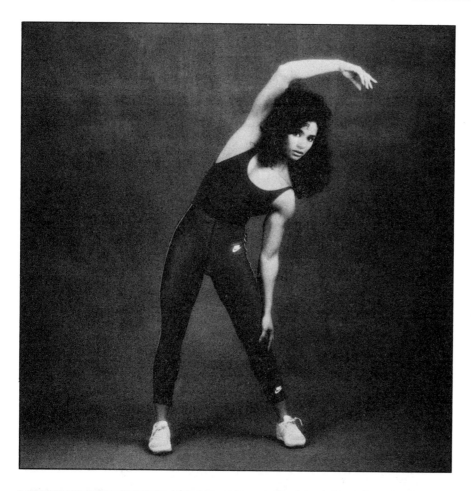

SIDE STRETCH (START)

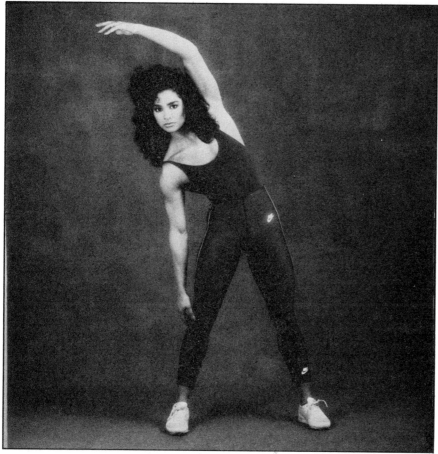

SIDE STRETCH (FINISH)

FLOOR TOUCH

This stretch pulls out the hamstrings and stretches the shoulder and triceps areas.

DIRECTIONS

- Stand with your legs shoulder width apart.

MOVEMENT

- Lean forward and place the palm of your right hand on the floor next to your left toe. (If you can't touch the floor, reach as far as you can; flexibility improves with effort.) Hold for 5 seconds. Repeat the movement with your left hand and right toe.

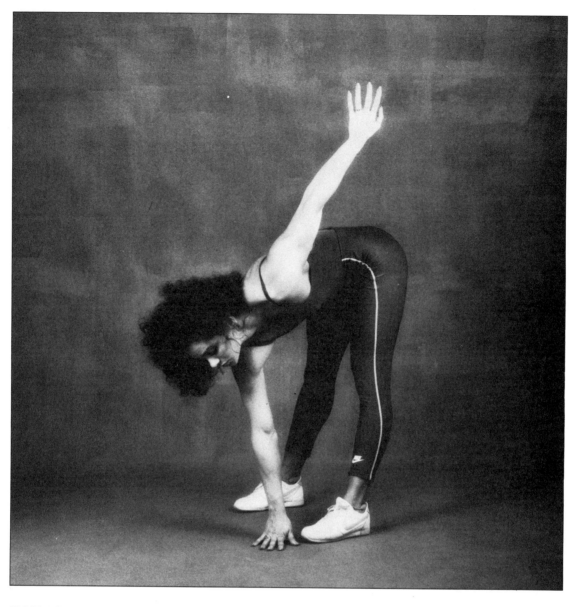

FLOOR TOUCH

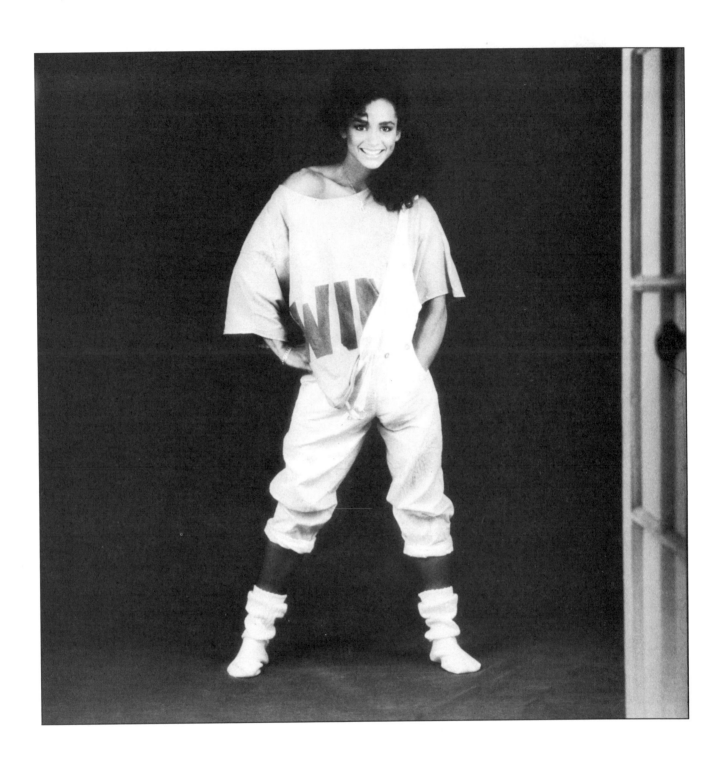

DIFFERENT WORKOUTS FOR DIFFERENT BODIES– FINDING YOURS

Your workout will depend upon the present condition of your body. We deliberately avoid categorizing our workouts by somatotypes such as endomorphic (fat or bulky), ectomorphic (slim with little body fat), and mesomorphic (muscular with little body fat). We do this because no matter what the present status of your body is, it will change after working out for a while.

If you are presently what we call a *bulky* body, you will slim down to an *in-between* body, and if you are a *slim* body, you will build up to an *in-between* body. All the women following our routine will appear to have nearly perfect bodies, and the fat percentage of their bodies should decrease to about 20 percent (when it may well be 35 percent now).

Traditionally, the mesomorphic body has been the coveted one, the one with lots of muscle and a low body fat percentage. But such categorization assumes that mesomorphic bodies are genetically inherited; we have discovered that no matter what your present body condition or your genetic endowment, you can reduce body fat and add shapely muscle. Eventually you will be close to what the physicians have termed the mesomorphic body.

Differently shaped bodies must begin with different routines. If you are an extremely overweight person, what we call a bulky body, it is necessary to use light weights and do high repetitions in order to burn off as much body fat as possible and at the same time build shapely muscles. If you are an extremely underweight person, what we call a slim body, it is necessary to use heavy weights and do fewer repetitions in order to build solid shapely muscles onto that frame which lacks mass. If you are neither overweight nor underweight, but just out of shape, it is necessary to use a combination of light and heavier weights and do a combination of high and low repetitions to burn fat and earn muscles.

Each of the three routines we have developed—bulky, slim, and in-between—work one body part at a time, working one half of the body on one day and the other half of the body on the next day. For example, no matter which category you fall into, you will ordinarily be working on your chest first, and you will be doing a certain number of exercises on your chest for about twenty minutes before you start on your shoulders. You will do exercises on your shoulders for twenty minutes and then move to your back for twenty minutes. Finally, you will work on your abdominals for about twenty minutes.

On the next training day you will begin by working on your biceps for twenty minutes, then you will work on your triceps for twenty minutes, then your legs, and finally your abdominals. As stated before, the abdominals must be trained every training day because they require additional stress in order to develop.

You will notice that some body parts respond very quickly to weights. Your chest and biceps will probably show some development after only three weeks training. Other body parts, such as the back and legs, take longer, but in time there will be a drastic change for the better (three to six months).

FINDING YOUR PRESENT BODY CONDITION

If we were to see you in a gym, we would tell you which workout to follow. In lieu of that, consult the charts below that take into account frame, height, and weight.

Check the Frame Determination Table first (p. 55) and follow the intructions for determining your frame. Then look up your height on the Height-Weight Chart (p. 56) and see if you are more than 10 pounds over the highest allowance for your height-frame. If so, you are a bulky body. If you are more than 10 pounds under the lowest weight allowance for your height-frame, then you are a slim body. If you are within the weight allowance for your height-frame, you are an in-between body.

Since this is not a book for competitive bodybuilders, we do not break our workouts down into beginning, intermediate, and advanced. Our workouts are designed to help you achieve the perfectly symmetrical, attractive hard body you desire, once and for all, now, and without a lot of technicalities.

The Height-Weight Chart is your guideline for deciding which body workout you will follow. First determine your frame:

Extend your arm and bend the forearm upward at a 90-degree angle. Keep your fingers straight and turn the inside of your wrist toward your body. Place your thumb and index finger of the other hand on the bones that protrude on each side of your elbow. Measure the space between your fingers against a ruler. Compare the results with the Frame Determination Table, which lists elbow measurements for medium-framed women. If your measurements are *lower* than those shown in the table, you are a *small-framed* woman. If your measurements are *higher* than those shown in the table you are *large-framed*, and if your measurements fall within the scale presented in the table, you are *medium-framed.* Note that height is measured in 1″ heels.

FRAME DETERMINATION TABLE

HEIGHT IN 1″ HEELS″	SPACE BETWEEN ELBOW BONES
4′ 10″–5′ 3″	2¼″–2½″
5′ 4″–5′ 11″	2⅜″–2⅝″
6′ 0″–	2½″–2¾″

SOURCE: Metropolitan Life Insurance Company (1983)

Now you are ready to look at the chart for your correct present body weight. Again, this chart is based on height in 1″ heels. The weight on the chart allows for 3 pounds of street clothing. For example, if you are 5 feet tall with a medium frame (as determined by the elbow bone width measurement) your present weight should be between 113 and 126 pounds. If you are more than 10 pounds less than 113 (that is, if you are 103 or less), you should do the slim body workout. If you are more than 10 pounds over the highest allowance of the chart, 126 (that is to say, if you are 137 or more), you should use the bulky body workout.

Most of you will be in the in-between category. Some women fall into the in-between category but feel fat or bulky. If this is the case, by all means follow the bulky body workout in order to trim fat faster and get down to a comfortable size. The chart is a guideline, and only you can determine the actual situation of your body.

If you are an in-between who feels skinny, follow the slim body workout in order to put on size more quickly. When you feel as if you are an in-between body, then you may move over to the in-between workout.

After you have been working out for a while, the charts will not be of use to you. As stated before, muscle weighs more than fat, so chances are you will

HEIGHT-WEIGHT CHART

HEIGHT*		SMALL	MEDIUM	LARGE
FEET	INCHES	FRAME	FRAME	FRAME
4	10	102–111	109–121	118–131
4	11	103–113	111–123	120–134
5	0	104–115	113–126	122–137
5	1	106–118	115–129	125–140
5	2	108–121	118–132	128–143
5	3	111–124	121–135	131–147
5	4	114–127	124–138	134–151
5	5	117–130	127–141	137–156
5	6	120–133	130–144	140–159
5	7	123–136	133–147	143–163
5	8	126–139	136–150	146–167
5	9	129–142	139–153	149–170
5	10	132–145	142–156	152–173
5	11	135–148	145–159	155–176
6	0	138–151	148–162	158–179

SOURCE: Metropolitan Life Insurance Company (1983)
* in 1″ heels

weigh more than a friend who is the same height as you and looks fatter than you do. People who work out tend to be within the allowed chart weight range for their height and frame even after working out for a year. The reason for this is quite obvious if you look at the wide weight range allowance. But after working out a year, you will not be much concerned about your weight range; what will concern you from now on will not be how much you weigh but what you see in the mirror.

The basic means of evaluating your body is the Height-Weight Chart. Even without the chart, however, there are obvious signs that make it clear to you what category you belong in. You will see that these signs fit in with what you have determined from the Height-Weight Chart.

BULKY BODY

You are obviously overweight, and knew it even before you found out by consulting the Height-Weight Chart. All past efforts to lose weight have resulted ultimately in additional weight gain. You don't believe that there's any hope for you.

SLIM BODY

You are obviously underweight, appear frail and weak, and have no visible muscular development. Most of your life people have told you you look skinny and have tried to feed you to get you up to par. You've tried eating and stuffing yourself, but nothing works.

IN-BETWEEN BODY

You look fine in clothing. In a bathing suit, however, your stomach bulges, showing lines of fat when you sit down, and you have fat pockets on your hips and just under your buttocks. Your arms may be sagging a bit in the triceps area and your skin is a bit too soft because of the thin layer of fat which is deposited beneath it. You are well within the correct weight range for your height, and others don't understand why you bother to diet. But you know that you are out of shape. You have tried running or other activities, but nothing seems to help. You have tried dieting also, but this does not change the shape of your body nor does it make the soft, flabby parts hard. You notice some fat piled upon fat on your legs (cellulite), and you wonder if it is really because you're getting older, even though you may not be much more than twenty-three.

CONCLUSION

Most of you will end up using the in-between body workout after a while. Some women, however, tend to be very slim, and they remain on the slim body workout because they continually want to put on body mass. No problem. They simply follow the slim body workout indefinitely and continually make progress. Bulky bodies, however, do go down in size and go into the in-between body workout.

The in-between workout is basically a lifetime maintenance program. Coupled with good eating habits (see Chapter Ten) the in-between body workout will guarantee you a perfectly shaped, sensual body for life.

Now that you have determined the present status of your body by the Height-Weight Chart and the above descriptions, it is time to learn what your particular routine will entail. Follow the description for your present body condition: *Chapter Six: The In-Between Body Workout,* or *Chapter Seven: The Slim Body Workout,* or *Chapter Eight: The Bulky Body Workout.*

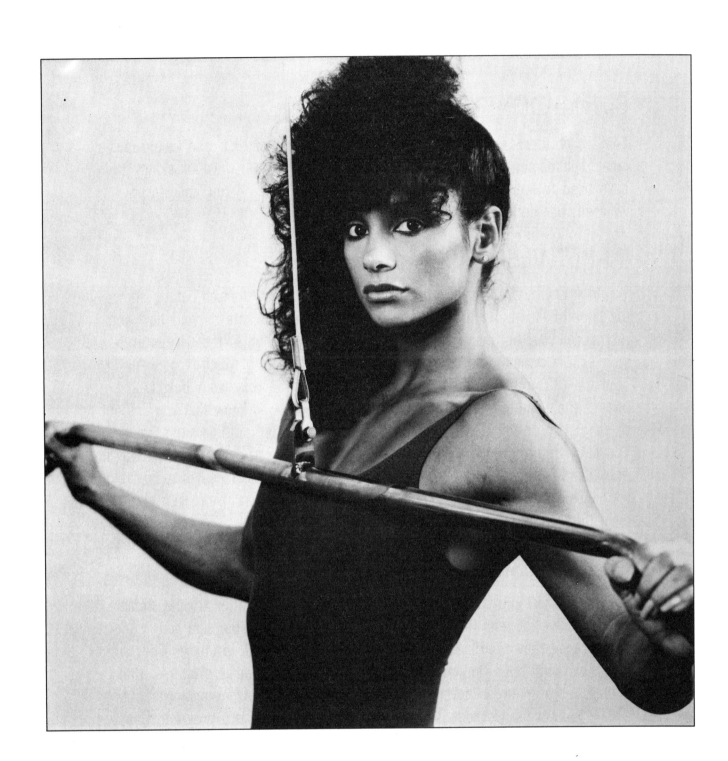

THE IN-BETWEEN BODY WORKOUT

It is possible to be just the right weight for one's height and look beautiful in street clothing but at the same time be out of shape and less than desirable in a bathing suit. In other words, there are many women who are not fat and not fit.

The key lies in the phrase *out of shape.* Some bodies have, over time, accumulated (through improper diet and lack of exercise) a great deal of cellulite (body fat bunched up into ripples), which can be eliminated with the Hard Bodies workout and intelligent dieting (explained in Chapter Ten).

After working out you may take the same dress size, but the body materials will have been reapportioned. Instead of having, for example, a 35 percent total body fat content, you'll get down to 20 or 25 percent. Your body will look better because it will be made up of more firm muscle and less loose, soft fat. Your walk will be more energetic and controlled because of strengthened supportive muscles, and clothing will drape in an elegant fashion over shapely muscles that have replaced misshapen fat. Your fear of bathing suits will have been cured.

The principle behind the Hard Bodies in-between body workout involves both high repetitions with light weights and low repetitions with heavy weights. This method burns off excess body fat and at the same time promotes the growth of shapely muscles. The body experiences a transformation: it becomes lean and shapely. It gives up the spongy fat deposited just below the skin surface. It takes on the shapely appearance of a sensual hard body.

BEGINNING THE WORKOUT

- Complete 3 sets of 8–15 repetitions for each exercise.
- There are 4 exercises for each body part, with the exception of legs, for which there are 5, and abdominals, for which there are 6.
- There are 12 sets for each body part, with the exception of legs (15) and abdominals (18).
- You will do chest, shoulders, back, and abdominals on one training day.
- You will do triceps, biceps, legs, and abdominals on the next training day.
- You will train 4 days a week, working each part of the body twice a week, except for the abdominals, which you will work 4 times a week.

HOW TO DETERMINE YOUR BEGINNING WEIGHT

Each exercise will involve different equipment (dumbbells, barbells, pulleys, machines, etc.) and will stress various muscles. Therefore, each requires different weight. Determine your beginning weight for each exercise by the following method:

- Select a light weight.
- Perform 15 repetitions with that weight.
- Add 2–10 pounds to that weight and perform 10–12 repetitions for your second set.
- Add 2–10 pounds to that weight for the third and final set and perform 6–8 repetitions.

NOTE: The idea is to combine high weights and low reps with high reps and low weights. So be sure to increase your weight enough with each set to the point that 15 reps becomes too difficult to complete. If you can reach 15 reps on the second set, your beginning weight was set too light.

PYRAMIDING

As discussed before, pyramiding is the most efficient way in which to add muscle mass to your body while eliminating excess body fat. The first set must be performed with a light enough weight to complete 15 repetitions with some effort but not a struggle. The second set must be heavy enough so that it is difficult to perform 12 repetitions. The third set must be heavy enough to make it difficult to reach 6 to 8 repetitions.

Using the example of the bench press, your first set will consist of 15 repetitions at 30 pounds. Your second set will be 10–12 repetitions at 40 pounds, and your final set will be 6–8 repetitions at 50 pounds.

How does one tell whether or not the weight is too light? If the weight is too light, you'll find it easy to get the 15 repetitions on your first set and the 12 and 8 repetitions on your second and third sets. Don't cheat yourself—raise the weight on your first set and each set following. If you cheat by keeping the weight lighter than is necessary, you will not see progress. You must continually challenge the muscle and work hard. Remember: no hard work, no hard body.

PERFORMING THE EXERCISES

Do each exercise in the following manner: Complete 3 sets of each exercise. For the first set do 15 repetitions, for the second set do 10–12 repetitions, and for the third set do 6–8 repetitions. Raise the weight on each set, utilizing the principle of pyramiding. When the weight of the beginning set becomes too easy, raise the weight of the first set and of each succeeding set. For example:

CHEST ROUTINE

Bench Press	Set 1.	30 pounds, 15 repetitions
	Set 2.	40 pounds, 10–12 repetitions
	Set 3.	50 pounds, 6–8 repetitions
Cable Crossover	Set 1.	5 pounds, 15 repetitions
	Set 2.	7½ pounds, 10–12 repetitions
	Set 3.	10 pounds, 6–8 repetitions
Incline Flye	Set 1.	10 pounds, 15 repetitions
	Set 2.	12 pounds, 10–12 repetitions
	Set 3.	15 pounds, 6–8 repetitions
And so on.		

Remember, after a few weeks the beginning weight will become too light. You must add weight to the first set and each succeeding set. If you do not, there will be no progress.

RAISING THE BEGINNING WEIGHT IN A WEEK OR TWO

After a few weeks (maybe less, maybe more—even as long as a month or two, but unlikely) your beginning weight will become too easy. This will happen because your muscles have grown stronger and larger. Using the bench press example, the beginning weight of 30 pounds will be so easy that the weight seems to fly up when you push it. You then increase your beginning weight to 40 pounds. Your second set will be 50 pounds at 10 repetitions and your final set will be 60 pounds at 8 repetitions.

The more you find yourself changing your beginning weight, the stronger you are getting. Your progress in a few months will surprise you. Some women have made as much as 30 to 40 pounds progress in three months time. But don't rush it. As long as your muscles are working to perform the exercise, they are growing because they are being forced to work. When you know the exercises are too easy, but you don't raise your beginning weight, your shape will not improve.

RESTING

The usual rest between sets is 30 seconds. You may want to rest only about 15 seconds between the first and second set because your first set involves light weight and high repetitions, but if you need a 30-second rest, take it. You may want to use the full 30 seconds in preparation for your second set, because the weight is a little heavier. You may take, if you need it, a 45-second rest between your second and third set because the weight will be still heavier.

Do not feel obliged to rest if you don't need it. As long as you are performing the exercises carefully, you may go as fast as you wish.

AEROBIC REQUIREMENT

In addition to doing your in-between body workout, we want you to perform an aerobic activity for one half hour, four days a week. This will help to burn excess body fat and condition your heart and lungs. You may run, ride the stationary bicycle, jump rope, or swim. Take as long as two months to get up to 30 minutes, starting the activity with 5 minutes the first week, 10 the second, and so on, until you reach the full 30 minutes. The importance of this aerobic activity cannot be overemphasized. Just because you are not outright fat does not mean that you can skip this. Your skin tone and body fat level—as well as your heart and lungs—demand this stimulation. (You will also be allowed more delicious food because you will be burning up calories.) Fit the aerobics in any time you can, before the gym workout, after it, on your gym days off and one gym day on, whatever is convenient for you. Some women ride a stationary bicycle while watching television. Others warm up by running around the gym for a half hour before starting to work out.

FINE-TUNING

At some point—usually after about 2 months—you may want to turn to Chapter Nine and follow the instructions for zeroing in on troublesome body parts. You may have big buttocks or saddlebags on your hips. Your stomach may be protruding and your legs may be too big for your upper body. This section tells you how to begin "bombing" that area with extra exercises and floor exercises.

You may not want to get involved in extra work at two months. Wait as long as six months if you choose. Your in-between body workout will be hitting these troublesome areas anyway and you will be making progress. In time, the "eyesores" will disappear, but the sooner you bomb them, the sooner they will go.

BREAKING IN

Do only 1 set of each exercise on your first training day. For example, instead of completing 3 sets of the bench press, do 1 set and move to the next exercise, the cable crossover. Perform only 1 set. Then move to the next exercise, the incline flye.

You will do the same breaking-in light workout on your second training day, when you do biceps, triceps, and legs. Only 1 set per exercise instead of the eventual 3 sets.

Remain at this pace for the first week. You will have trained four times that first week, twice for each body part (four times for abdominals).

By your second week you are ready to do 2 sets per exercise. Do this for each exercise for the entire four days of training this second week.

By your third week you are ready to do your full workout of 3 sets per exercise. Now you can follow the prescribed instructions exactly. Your muscles will have been broken in gently.

Some ambitious women want to start out with all 3 sets per exercise right away. Don't. It results in undue soreness and a temptation to quit. You'll feel the effects even starting slowly.

The full routine should take about 90 minutes.

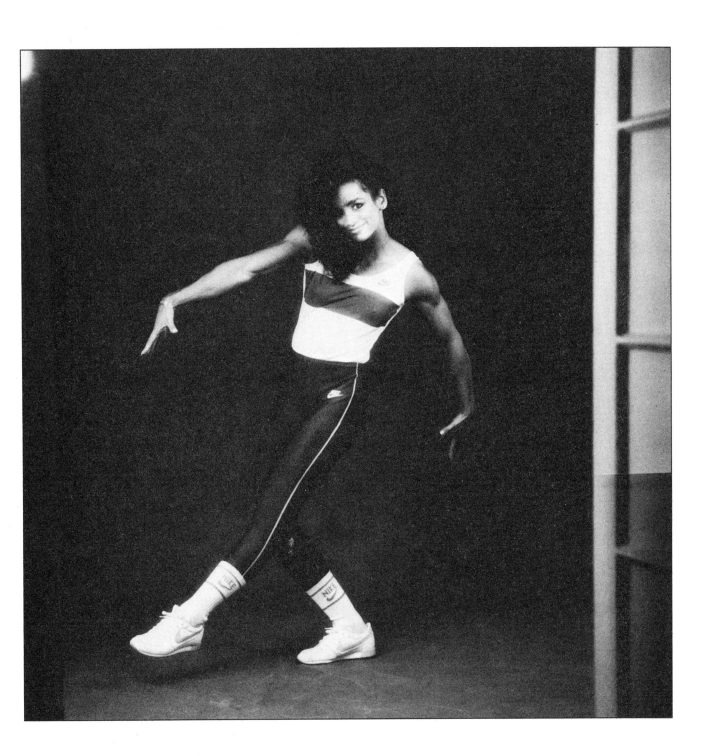

CHEST ROUTINE

FLAT BENCH PRESS

This exercise works the pectoral muscles (breast area) of the chest. It can be done on the Universal Gym, on the Nautilus, or with free weights.

DIRECTIONS	• Lie on the bench with your shoulders just under the bar of the press. • Grip the bar or the pressing handles about shoulder width apart.
MOVEMENT	• Hold on to the bar and slowly lower it to your chest. • Slowly raise the bar to starting position. • Repeat the movement until you have performed the correct number of repetitions for your set.
SUGGESTIONS	Vary the grip every week, making it a bit narrower than shoulder width and then a bit wider; this ensures that every area of the pectorals (breast area) is worked.
DON'TS	Do not let the bar "fall" on the downward movement. Control the weight at all times. There is a greater tendency to "drop" the weight when using a machine. Don't let this happen.

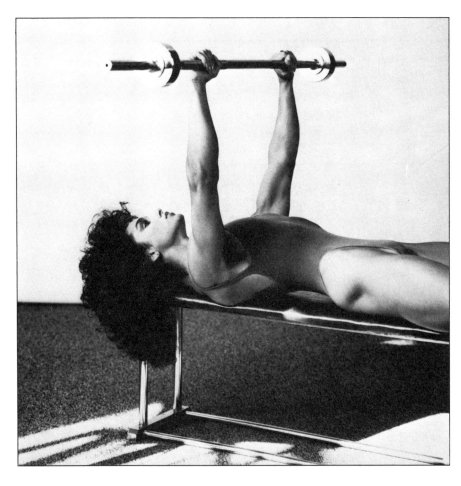

FLAT BENCH PRESS (START)

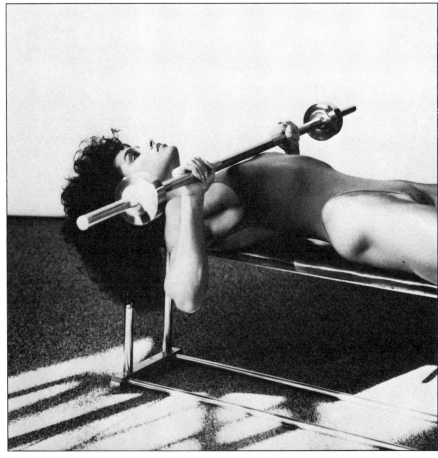

FLAT BENCH PRESS (FINISH)

CABLE CROSSOVER

This exercise develops the pectoral area of the chest, especially the inner and lower areas.

DIRECTIONS	• Take one handle of the crossover pulley machine in each hand and stand in the middle of the workout area with your feet apart in a natural position, facing the mirror if there is one.
	• Hold your arms, pulleys in hands, upward at 45-degree angles, arms slightly bent and hands facing downward.
	• Bend forward slightly from the waist, with feet firmly planted, and begin the movement.
MOVEMENT	• Pull the handles downward, slowly, in an arc as you flex (tighten and squeeze together) your pectoral (chest) muscles.
	• Bring the handles down until they cross each other in the center of your body, wrist over wrist, and hold for one second.
	• Slowly, controlling the weights at all times, allow your arms to ascend to starting position and immediately repeat the movement until you have performed the correct number of repetitions for your set.
SUGGESTIONS	Work one arm at a time if you find yourself favoring one over the other.
DON'TS	Never let the weight control you or jerk you upward as you return to starting position. Concentrate at all times.

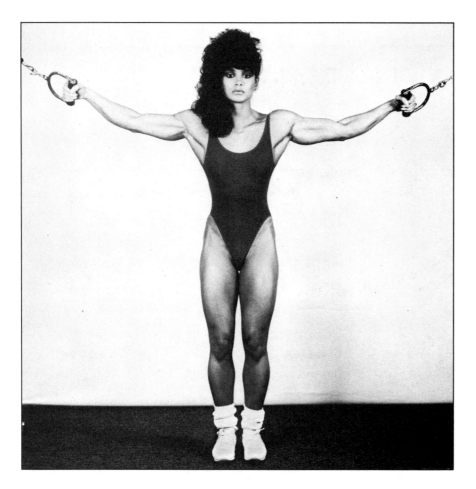

CABLE CROSSOVER (START)

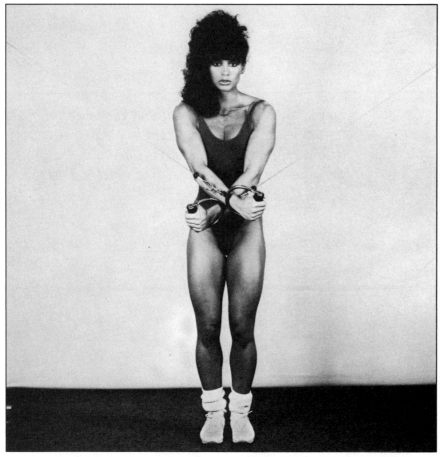

CABLE CROSSOVER (FINISH)

INCLINE FLYE

This exercise develops the pectoral (breast) area of the chest, especially the upper chest muscles, and slightly develops the front deltoid (shoulder muscle).

DIRECTIONS

- Lie on an incline bench with one dumbbell in each hand.

- Extend your arms over your head so that the dumbbells are held just above your shoulder joints at full arm's length. (Be sure that your palms are facing inward at all times.)

MOVEMENT

- Slowly move the dumbbells outward and downward in a semicircle on each side, moving them outward until you feel a full stretch in the chest area.

- Trace the same arc back to starting position and repeat the movement until you have performed the correct number of repetitions for your set.

SUGGESTIONS

As you are moving the weights to the outer position, be sure to expand your chest, stretching it as much as possible. When you are returning to starting position, squeeze and flex your chest as much as possible.

DON'TS

Do not raise yourself by arching your back when performing the movement. If you find yourself unable to control this temptation, perhaps the weights are too heavy. Your back should remain flatly on the bench at all times. Concentrate. Control the weights.

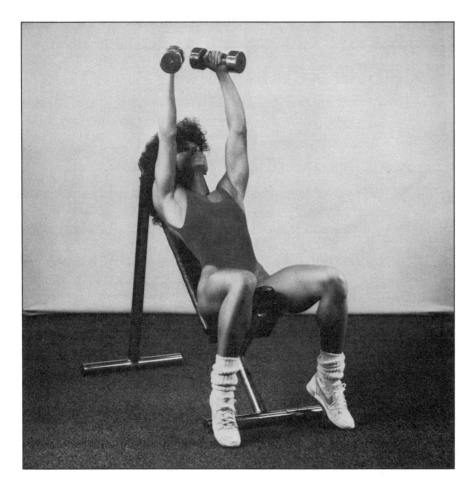

INCLINE FLYE (START)

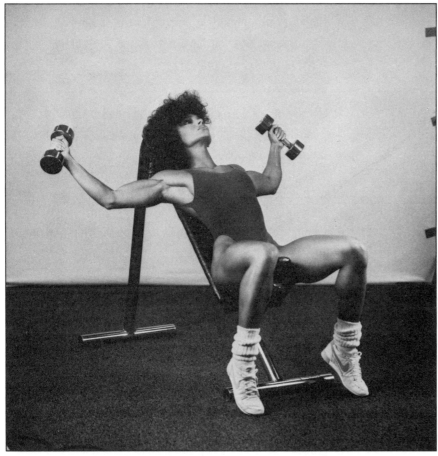

INCLINE FLYE (FINISH)

CROSS BENCH PULLOVER

This exercise develops the entire pectoral (breast) area and works the serratus (side muscle) and latissimi dorsi (back muscles).

DIRECTIONS	• Hold a dumbbell with both hands so that your palms are against the inside plate of the dumbbell and your thumbs are touching. • Lean over a flat exercise bench (or the specially curved one if there is one) so that your shoulders touch the edge of the bench. • Extend your arms upward, placing the dumbbell straight above your neck, and with feet slightly apart and knees bent, prepare to begin.
MOVEMENT	• Slowly lower the dumbbell over the bench, behind you, going as low as possible and getting a full stretch in the pectoral area. (The dumbbell will be moving in a semi-circle directly behind your head.) • Raise the dumbbell to starting position and repeat the movement until you have performed the correct number of repetitions for your set.
SUGGESTIONS	If you are using a rounded bench you will be placing your feet astride the bench and your back along the rounded part of the bench. The actual pullover will be done over the curved part of the bench. Whichever bench you use, be sure to stretch your chest as much as possible as you lower the weight to its lowest possible point. As you raise the weight to starting position, be sure to flex (squeeze together) your chest muscles.
DON'TS	Do not simply "drop" the weight down and "lurch" it back up to starting position. Such poor technique will result in small and injured muscles. Concentrate.

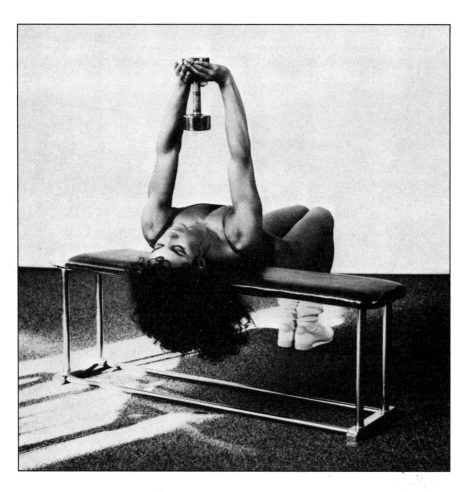

CROSS BENCH PULLOVER
(START)

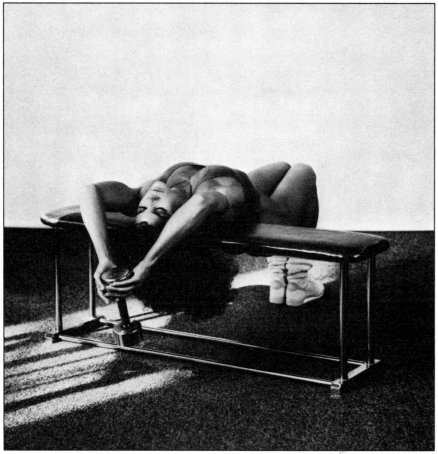

CROSS BENCH PULLOVER
(FINISH)

SHOULDER ROUTINE

SIDE INCLINE LATERAL

This exercise develops the front deltoid (shoulder muscle) and helps to develop the trapezius (the muscle located between the shoulder and the neck).

DIRECTIONS	• Lie sideways on a low incline bench, holding a dumbbell in your right hand, palm down and thumb facing down. • Bend your elbow to a 90-degree angle. (You are lying on your left side.)
MOVEMENT	• Slowly raise your upper right arm in a hingelike manner until your elbow is in line with your shoulder. • Pause for a split second and slowly return to starting position and immediately repeat the movement until you have completed the correct number of repetitions for your set. • Repeat for your other arm while lying on your right side.
SUGGESTIONS	Use a light weight and do the exercise in a very strict fashion. Concentrate on the shoulder area as you raise and lower your elbow, flexing your shoulder muscles at all times.
DON'TS	Do not jerk the weight up and never let it drop down to starting position. Slowly raise and lower it, controlling the movement at all times. Picture your deltoid taking shape and gaining definition.

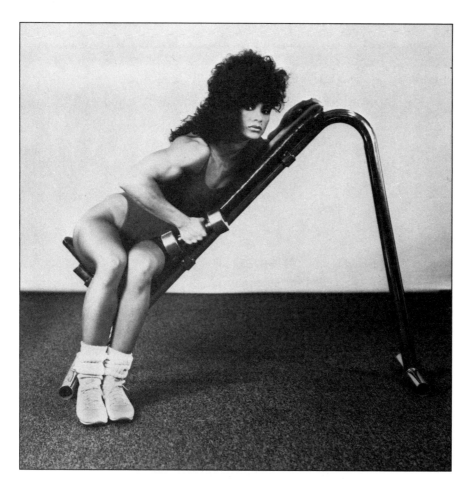

SIDE INCLINE LATERAL
(START)

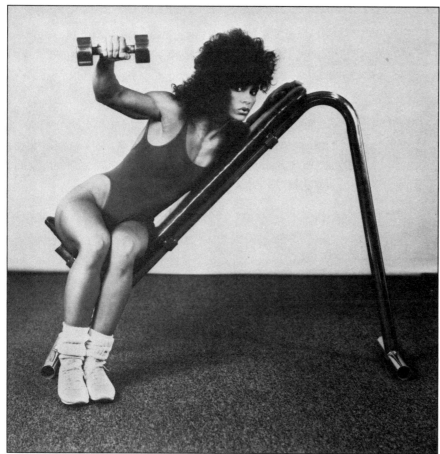

SIDE INCLINE LATERAL
(FINISH)

MILITARY PRESS TO THE FRONT

This exercise develops the deltoids (shoulder muscles) and also the trapezius. It may be done with a barbell, on a Nautilus or Universal Gym machine, or on a freestanding machine. The description below applies to a freestanding machine.

DIRECTIONS

- Sit on the machine stool, facing the machine.

- With palms facing away from you, grip the machine handles in the center of each handle.

MOVEMENT

- Slowly extend your arms straight upward, controlling the weight at all times, until your arms are fully extended upward.

- Return to starting position (your elbows should just about touch your sides).

- Repeat this movement until you have performed the correct number of repetitions for your set.

SUGGESTIONS

If you decide to do this exercise with a barbell, you may stand and perform the movement with your legs shoulder width apart. Be sure to begin with light weight.

DON'TS

Do not jerk the handles upward and then let them "drop" back to starting position. Control the weight at all times. Do not rest when you return to starting position, but rather immediately begin the next repetition.

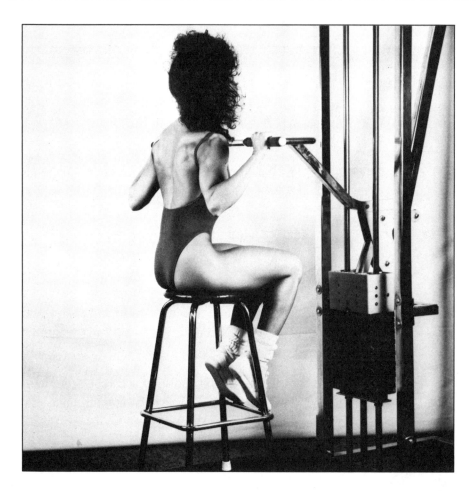

**MILITARY PRESS
TO THE FRONT (START)**

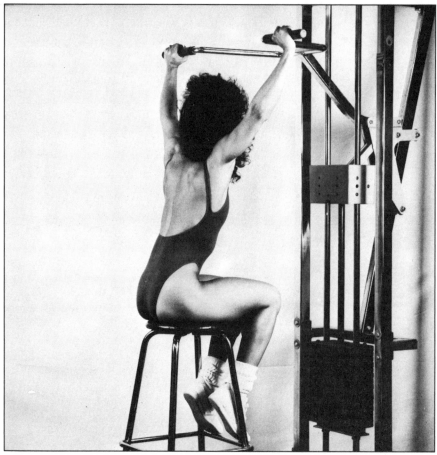

**MILITARY PRESS
TO THE FRONT (FINISH)**

SIDE LATERAL RAISE

This exercise develops the front and side deltoids (shoulder muscles) and helps to develop the trapezius.

DIRECTIONS	• Hold one dumbbell in each hand in front of you, with the dumbbells touching each other at the center of your body.
	• With elbows slightly bent and held about waist high, lean slightly forward.
MOVEMENT	• Slowly raise the dumbbells outward toward your sides, forming a semicircle on each side until you reach your shoulders on each side.
	• Slowly return to starting position and repeat the movement until you have performed the correct number of repetitions for your set.
SUGGESTIONS	If you wish to develop your trapezius with this exercise, raise the dumbbells to your ears rather than just to your shoulders. Your shoulders will still be developed, but not as much because you are now putting more stress on the trapezius (the muscle between your shoulder and neck).
DON'TS	Never swing the weight up and drop it down. Slowly raise and lower the weight while contracting your shoulder muscles and concentrating on the shoulder area. If you find that you cannot avoid swinging the weight, it is too heavy. Go lighter.

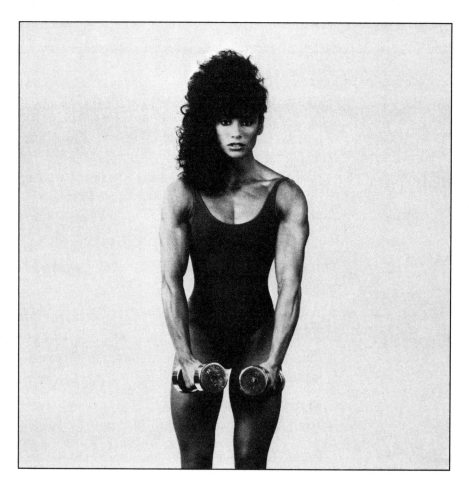

SIDE LATERAL RAISE (START)

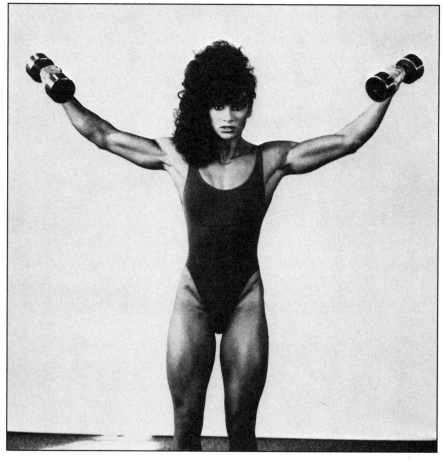

SIDE LATERAL RAISE (FINISH)

UPRIGHT ROW

This exercise works the deltoid and the trapezius areas of the shoulder.

DIRECTIONS

- Hold a barbell with your thumbs 7 inches apart and facing down with the palms of your hands facing your body.

- Lower the barbell so that your arms are hanging down at your sides and the barbell is leaning against your upper thighs.

MOVEMENT

- Slowly pull the barbell up until it almost touches your chin. (Be sure to keep your elbows high while pulling the barbell upward.)

- When the barbell reaches your chin, flex your shoulders and then slowly lower the barbell to starting position.

- Repeat the movement until you have performed the correct number of repetitions for your set.

SUGGESTIONS

Change your grip from time to time, taking a wider then a narrower grip about every week and a half. This will ensure your working every part of the shoulder area.

As you raise and lower the barbell, picture the muscles contracting and expanding. Remember how the muscles look on the anatomy chart (pp. 12–13) and mentally see them growing and becoming more defined.

DON'TS

Do not jerk the weight up and let it drop down. Be sure that you feel your shoulders and not your arms doing the work.

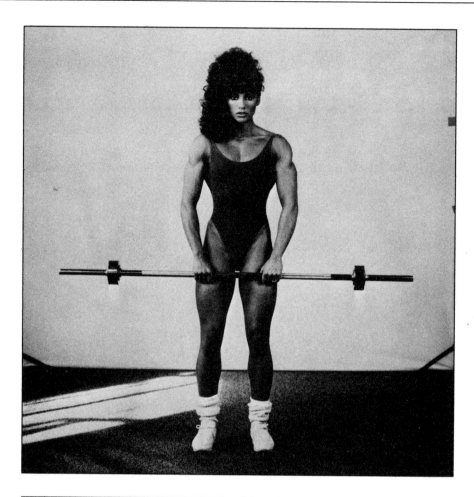

UPRIGHT ROW (START)

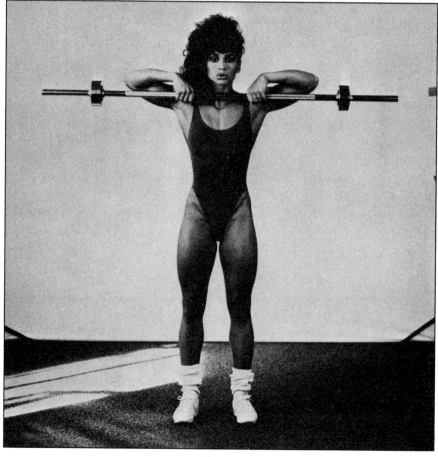

UPRIGHT ROW (FINISH)

BACK ROUTINE

SHRUG

This exercise develops the trapezius muscles of your upper back (connecting your neck to your shoulders). A shrug can be done on a Nautilus machine, on a Universal Gym machine, or with a simple barbell. It is described here for the barbell.

DIRECTIONS

- Stand in front of a mirror with a barbell held in front of your thighs, arms extended down.

- Place your feet a natural width apart and stand in an upright position.

MOVEMENT

- Slowly raise your shoulders as high as possible and rotate them backwards and downwards in a shrugging motion.

- Repeat this movement until you have performed the correct number of repetitions for your set.

SUGGESTIONS

Be sure to get a full stretch on the downward movement of the shrug. Remember to rotate your shoulders as far back as possible. A 45-pound barbell should be comfortable.

DON'TS

Never cut the movement short. Do a full shrug. Do not lose concentration, but fully rotate your shoulder muscles when doing the exercise.

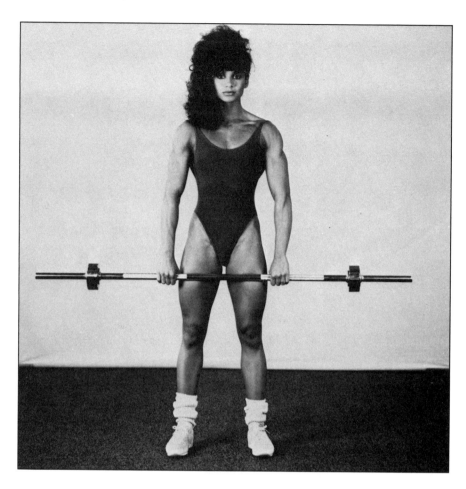

SHRUG (START)

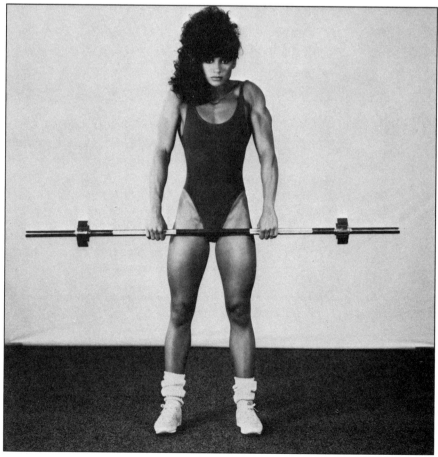

SHRUG (FINISH)

SEATED PULLEY ROW

This exercise works the latissimi dorsi (lats), the muscles of the upper back. It will widen your back and help create the aesthetically appealing V shape, the look possessed by so many athletes.

DIRECTIONS

- Take hold of the floor pulley bar, palms facing down, and seat yourself with your legs slightly bent and your feet supported by the metal foot-rest bar.
- Extend your arms completely and lean forward as far as possible.

MOVEMENT

- Pull the handles toward your chest, while at the same time you bend your arms and straighten your back. (Be careful to keep your body in an upright, perpendicular position. It will be tempting to lean backwards.)

- Touch your upper abdomen with the handles and push out your chest as far as you can, feeling the crunch in your back. (Remember to keep your upper arms close to your body while pulling in.)

- Return to starting position and repeat the movement until you have completed the correct number of repetitions for your set.

SUGGESTIONS

This exercise provides a natural stretch for the back, so if your back is a little stiff, start your back routine with this exercise. Remember to stretch as far forward as possible each time you return to starting position and to allow your back to stretch fully. Picture the muscles on the sides of your back expanding and forming themselves into a V.

DON'TS

Do not let the weight sweep you forward on the return position, but rather slowly return to starting position, controlling the weight at all times.

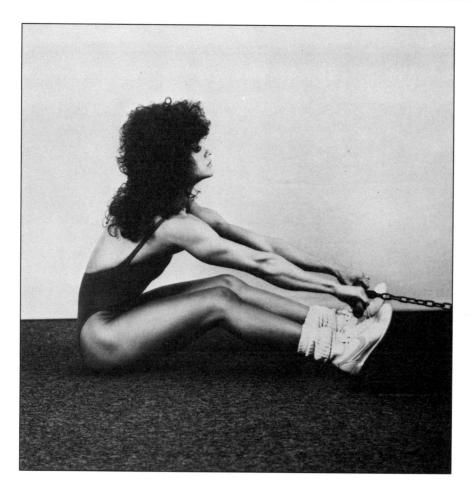

SEATED PULLEY ROW
(START)

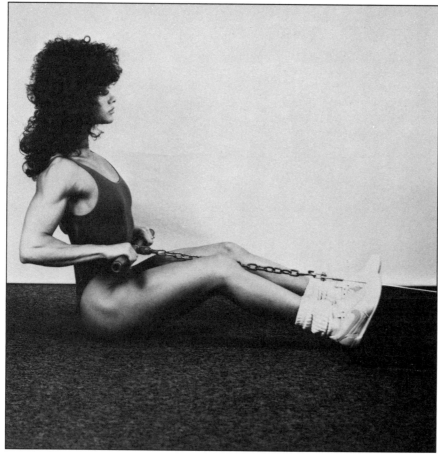

SEATED PULLEY ROW
(FINISH)

DUMBBELL BENT ROW

This exercise works your latissimi dorsi (back lat) muscles. It helps to widen your back, creating that appealing V look coveted by bodybuilders and models. It also adds shape to the back.

DIRECTIONS

- Support yourself over an exercise bench with your right hand and right knee.

- Take hold of a dumbbell in your left hand and let your left arm hang down in a straight line with your shoulder joint.

MOVEMENT

- Pull the dumbbell up to your waist slowly while moving your hip slightly to cooperate with the exercising arm.

- Control the weight as you slowly lower it to starting position.

- Repeat the movement until you have completed the correct number of repetitions for your set.

- Switch to the other arm and perform the correct number of repetitions for the set.

SUGGESTIONS

When you have reached the lower (starting) position, be sure to let the weight pull you into a stretch.

DON'TS

Do not let the weight fall as you lower it. Control the weight at all times, concentrating on the lat.

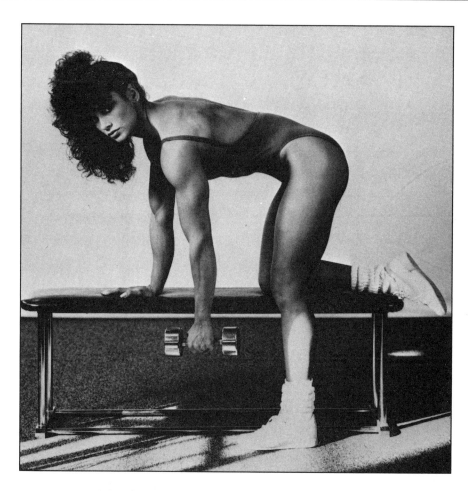

DUMBBELL BENT ROW (START)

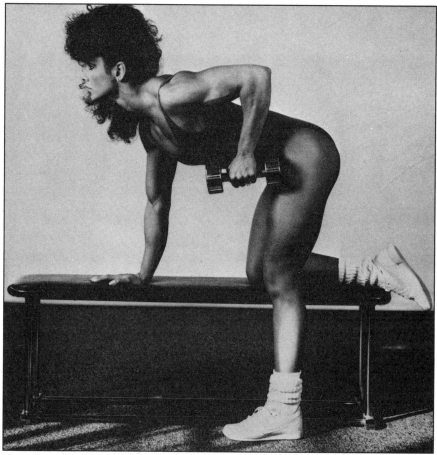

DUMBBELL BENT ROW (FINISH)

LAT MACHINE PULLDOWN TO THE FRONT

This exercise develops the latissimi dorsi muscles of your back. It can be done on the Universal Gym, the Nautilus, or a freestanding lat machine. We describe it for the freestanding lat machine, since most gyms have one.

DIRECTIONS

- Sit in the machine seat with your knees under the knee-restraining bar.

- Hold the lat machine bar in a shoulder-width grip with palms forward and thumbs up.

- Extend your arms upward in a ready position.

MOVEMENT

- Pull slowly downward on the bar, making sure you feel the stress in your lats (back muscles) rather than in your arms. (Squeeze your back as you pull.)

- Touch the bar to your upper chest and slowly return the bar to starting position, controlling it at all times.

- Repeat this movement until you have performed the correct number of repetitions for your set.

SUGGESTIONS

Concentrate continually on your back muscles, making sure that you feel the stress in your back and not your arms.

DON'TS

Do not let your arms do the work; if you do you will never see lat development. Doing the exercise incorrectly will result in years of wasted effort. Be sure to allow the weight to stretch your back upward on the return movement.

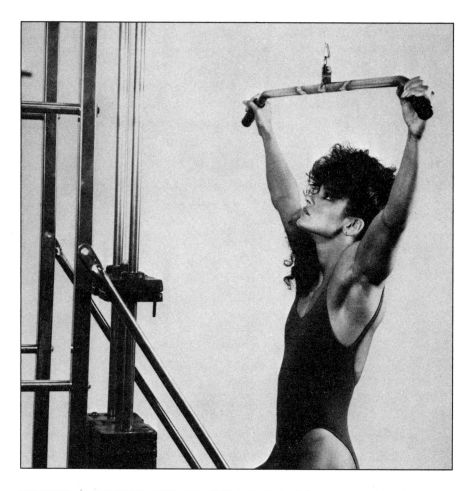

LAT MACHINE PULLDOWN
TO THE FRONT (START)

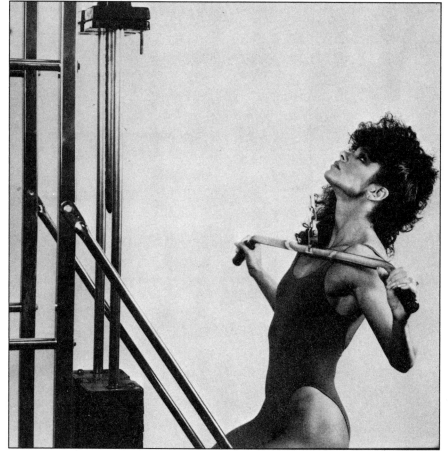

LAT MACHINE PULLDOWN
TO THE FRONT (FINISH)

BICEPS ROUTINE

INCLINE DUMBBELL CURL

This exercise develops the entire biceps area.

DIRECTIONS	• With a dumbbell in each hand, lie on an incline bench. • With palms upward and arms falling straight down, prepare to begin the movement.
MOVEMENT	• Keeping your upper arms close to your body, slowly raise the dumbbells (both at the same time) in a semicircular motion, until the dumbbells reach shoulder height. • Slowly return the dumbbells to starting position and repeat the movement until you have performed the correct number of repetitions to complete your set.
SUGGESTIONS	You may alternate right-left-right-left until you have completed a full set. Remember to flex your biceps on the upward movement. Watch your biceps move as it stretches out on the downward movement and crunches together on the upward movement. Concentrate. Flex. Squeeze.
DON'TS	Do not allow your back to rise from the incline bench in an effort to give yourself leverage to "jerk" the weights. If you find you are not able to keep yourself from rising off the bench, decrease the weight. This exercise must be done in strict form or no visible muscular development will result.

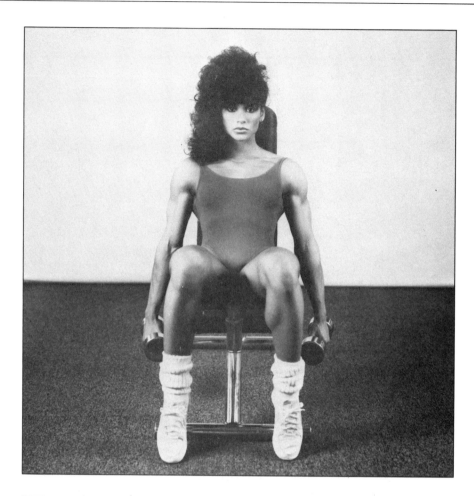

INCLINE DUMBBELL CURL
(START)

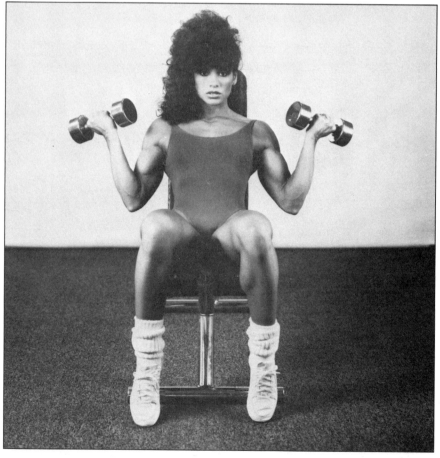

INCLINE DUMBBELL CURL
(FINISH)

STANDING BARBELL CURL

This exercise develops the entire biceps area.

DIRECTIONS	• With palms forward, hold the barbell with a shoulder-width grip (or a few inches wider) and rest the barbell against your upper thighs.
	• Stand in a natural position, upright, and keep your upper arms tightly pressed to your sides.
	• Let the barbell's weight fall fully on your arms, which are now fully extended downward.
MOVEMENT	• Slowly raise the barbell to your upper chest until it grazes your chin and slowly return to starting position.
	• When you reach starting position, slightly open your hands, letting the barbell hang loosely on your fingers for a split second.
	• Tighten your grip again and slowly raise the barbell, repeating the movement until you have completed the correct number of repetitions for your set.
SUGGESTIONS	Flex your biceps on the upward movement and get a full stretch on the downward movement.
DON'TS	Do not jerk the barbell upward and do not let it drop down to starting position. Control the weight at all times. Watch your biceps in the mirror as it contracts and expands.

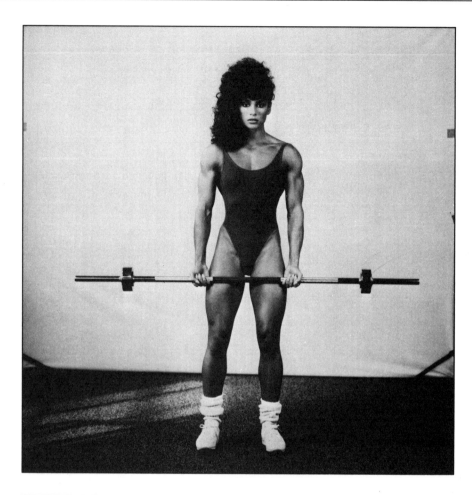

**STANDING BARBELL CURL
(START)**

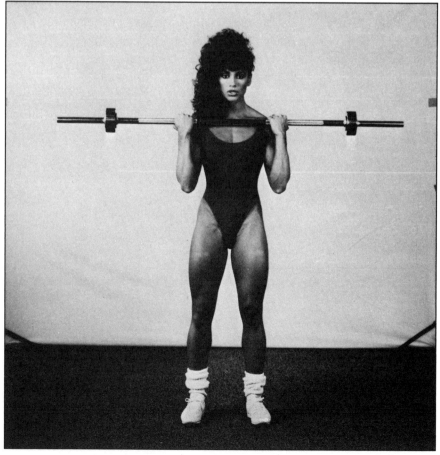

**STANDING BARBELL CURL
(FINISH)**

ONE-ARM PREACHER CURL

This exercise develops the entire biceps area, with a special emphasis on the lower portion of the muscle.

DIRECTIONS

- With a dumbbell in your right hand, lean over the preacher bench completely forward so that the edge of the bench is directly under your armpit.

- Keep your left arm relaxed at your side or resting on the bench and let your right arm with the dumbbell hang straight down, fully extended over the bench surface.

MOVEMENT

- Slowly raise your right arm, flexing your biceps and concentrating on the gradual movement of the biceps. Be sure to keep your wrist from bending back. Keep it straight.

- Raise the dumbbell all the way up until it grazes your chin.

- Slowly lower the dumbbell to starting position and repeat this movement until you have performed the correct number of repetitions for your set.

- Repeat the set for your left arm.

SUGGESTIONS

You must lean as hard as you can on the preacher bench in order to take the stress away from every part of the body except the biceps muscle.

DON'TS

Do not jerk the dumbbell on the upward movement or let it drop down as you lower it, but rather control it at all times. Concentrate on watching the biceps contract. Remember to squeeze and flex the muscle.

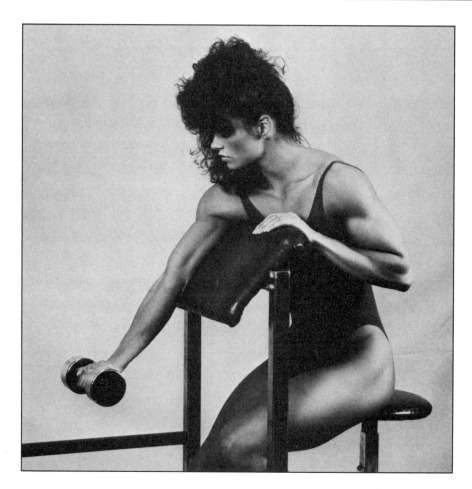

ONE-ARM PREACHER CURL
(START)

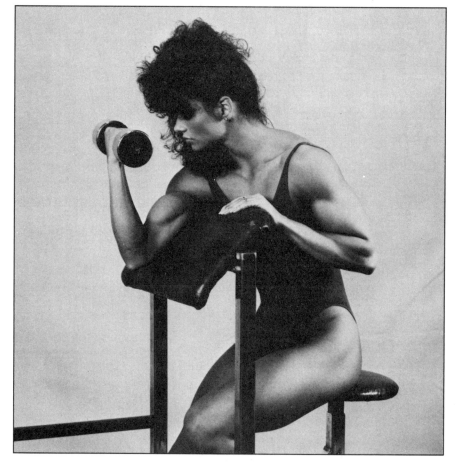

ONE-ARM PREACHER CURL
(FINISH)

PULLEY CURL

This exercise develops the entire biceps muscle. It may be performed on the Universal Gym or a freestanding pulley machine. Pulleys may be done with one or two arms at a time. We describe it for one arm because this method allows greater concentration.

DIRECTIONS

- Stand in front of the floor pulley and take hold of the handle with your right hand, palm facing upward. Relax your left arm.

- Stand with your feet shoulder width apart and keep your arms straight at your sides.

MOVEMENT

- Slowly raise your right arm in a semicircle until the pulley handle grazes your chin, and controlling the weight, return to starting position.

- Repeat this movement until you have done the correct number of repetitions for your set.

- Repeat the exercise for the left arm.

SUGGESTIONS

Remember to flex your biceps as you pull upward. Watch your biceps grow and stretch as you pull and lower the weight.

DON'TS

Do not use your back or torso to help you jerk the weight upward. Remember not to let your upper arms wander away from your body as you do the exercise. Concentrate.

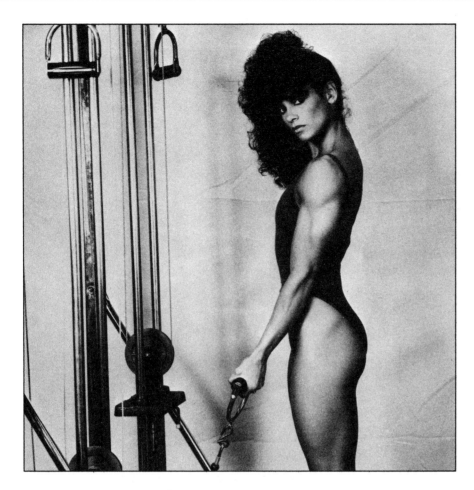

PULLEY CURL (START)

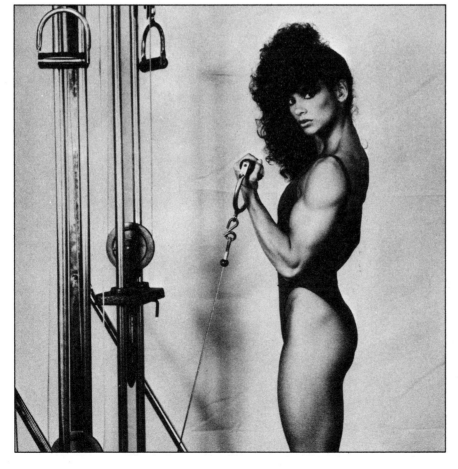

PULLEY CURL (FINISH)

TRICEPS ROUTINE

LYING TRICEPS EXTENSION

This exercise develops the entire triceps area.

DIRECTIONS	• With a barbell in your hands, lie on a flat exercise bench on your back. • Hold the barbell with palms facing upward and 7 inches apart. Your arms should be bent, and the barbell held just above your forehead. Bring your knees up and rest your feet on the bench.
MOVEMENT	• Slowly straighten your arms until the barbell is held directly above your eyes. • Slowly return to starting position and repeat this movement until you have performed the correct number of repetitions for your set.
SUGGESTIONS	You must vary your grip from time to time (about every week and a half). You may grip the bar with your hands anywhere from 3 to 8 inches apart.
DON'TS	Do not allow your shoulders to do the work. Keep your upper arms close to your body and concentrate on feeling the stress in your triceps area. Refer to the anatomy chart (pp. 12–13) continually and remember to picture *your* triceps working.

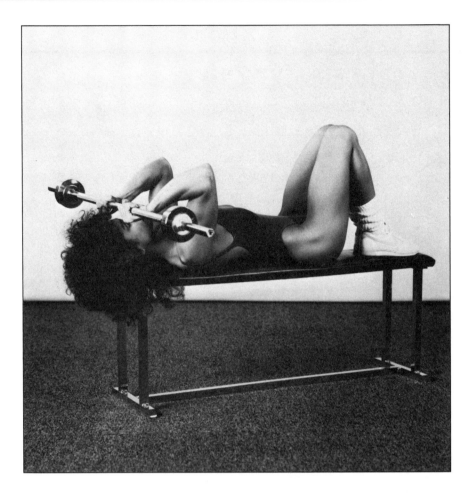

LYING TRICEPS EXTENSION
(START)

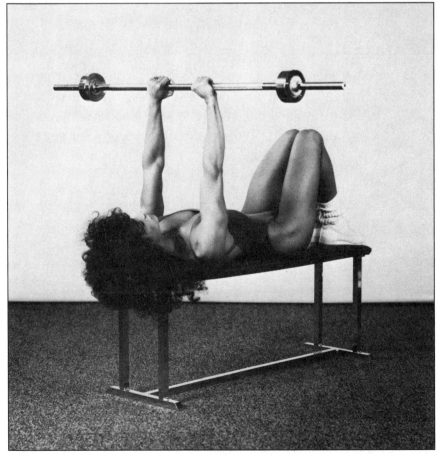

LYING TRICEPS EXTENSION
(FINISH)

DIP BETWEEN BENCHES

This exercise develops the entire triceps area.

DIRECTIONS	• Line up two flat exercise benches so that they are parallel to each other and wide enough apart so that when you lean on one with the palm of your hands, your heels are firmly placed on the far edge of the other. (The benches will be about 2–3 feet apart.)
	• Curl your fingers around the edge of the bench for support.
	• Your hands should be 5 inches apart.
MOVEMENT	• Lower your body slowly by bending your upper arms.
	• Go as low as you possibly can and then slowly return to starting position.
	• Repeat this movement until you have performed the correct number of repetitions for your set.
SUGGESTIONS	If you wish, perform this exercise first in your triceps workout because it provides a good stretch for those muscles.
DON'TS	Do not lower yourself a mere 2 or 3 inches. Go all the way. Bend your arms as much as possible, and after going as far down as you can, be sure to raise yourself until your arms are completely straight. Do not rest once you have returned to starting position. Keep on going until you complete your set. Concentrate.

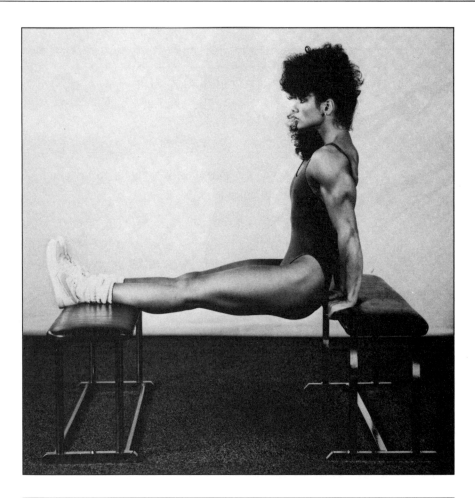

**DIP BETWEEN BENCHES
(START)**

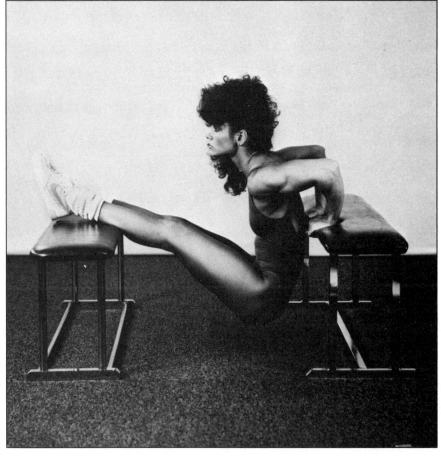

**DIP BETWEEN BENCHES
(FINISH)**

ONE-ARM DUMBBELL TRICEPS EXTENSION

This exercise emphasizes the inner and middle area of the triceps.

DIRECTIONS

- Stand in front of a mirror with a dumbbell in your left hand, in a natural position.

- Raise your left arm straight up so that your biceps is touching your ear. Hold the dumbbell so that the palm of your hand is facing the mirror. Place your right arm around your waist.

MOVEMENT

- Slowly lower the dumbbell so that it moves down behind your head and finally touches the back of your neck.

- Slowly return the weight to starting position and repeat this movement until you have performed the correct number of repetitions for your set.

- Repeat the set for your right arm. (Remember: you must do three sets on *each* arm, one for the left, then one for the right, and so on. Do not complete all three sets for one arm and then the other. Alternate sets.)

SUGGESTIONS

Be sure to hold the dumbbell securely at all times and to keep your triceps flexed (tightened) and your biceps close to the side of your head. The only movement is that of your forearm from the elbow joint.

DON'TS

Do not keep your nonworking hand on your shoulder near your neck. You may smash your fingers.

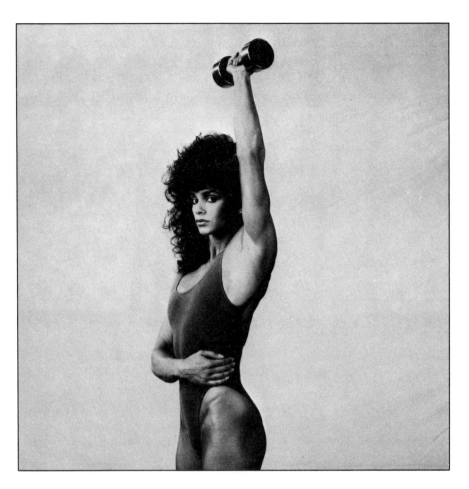

**ONE-ARM DUMBBELL
TRICEPS EXTENSION (START)**

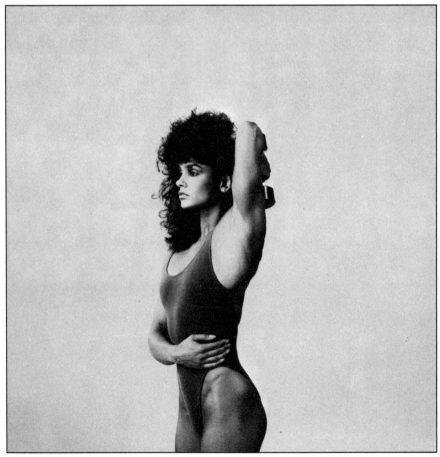

**ONE-ARM DUMBBELL
TRICEPS EXTENSION (FINISH)**

PULLEY PUSHDOWN

This exercise works the entire triceps area. It can be done on the Universal Gym or on a freestanding pulley.

DIRECTIONS	• Place the straight pulley pushdown bar on the pulley. • Hold the bar with your palms facing away from you, 6 inches apart. • Bending at the elbows, fully extend your forearms upward and keep your upper arms pinned to your body.
MOVEMENT	• Slowly lower the bar, bringing your forearms straight down. • Slowly return to starting position and repeat the movement until you have performed the correct number of repetitions for your set.
SUGGESTIONS	This exercise may be done with a curved bar or a straight bar. The curved bar, however, is not always available.
DON'TS	Do not allow your upper arms to leave their position (pinned to your sides). If your elbows are away from your body, you are not working your triceps but your shoulders—and that inefficiently. Concentrate and picture your triceps working. Remember the anatomy chart of the triceps.

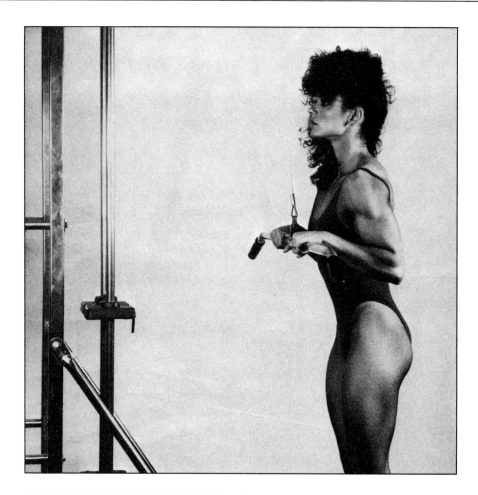

PULLEY PUSHDOWN (START)

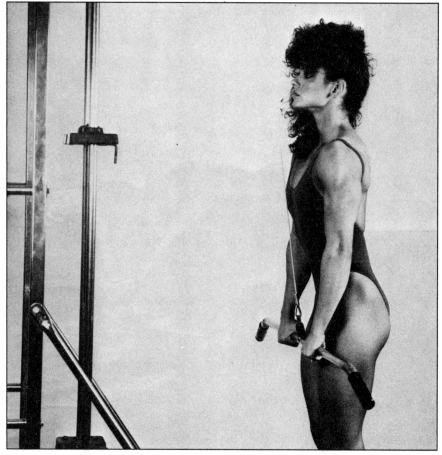

PULLEY PUSHDOWN (FINISH)

L E G   R O U T I N E

LUNGE

This exercise develops the muscles of the upper front quadriceps (thigh muscles) as well as the gluteus maximus (buttock muscles).

DIRECTIONS

- Place a barbell across your shoulders behind your neck, resting the barbell on your trapezius muscles. (No rubber pad or towel is needed. Do not rely on crutches.)

- Stand with your feet a natural width apart (about 6 inches) and be sure that your toes are pointing in a natural, straight-ahead position, ready to lunge.

MOVEMENT

- Keeping your right leg straight, step forward with your left foot as far as possible, bending your right knee as you do. (Keep your torso from leaning forward by looking straight ahead, preferably into a mirror.)

- Continue the movement until your left knee almost touches the floor and then slowly return to starting position.

- Repeat the movement for the right leg and continue this left–right movement until you have completed the correct number of repetitions for your set.

SUGGESTIONS

Be sure to stretch your quadriceps (thigh muscles) as you lunge forward. (You should feel the muscle pulling and stretching.) Some people prefer to lunge onto a block of wood in order to get a more complete stretch.

DON'TS

Do not shorten the distance of the lunge as you go along. Keep the lunge a full stretch, making sure to step as deeply as possible. Concentrate.

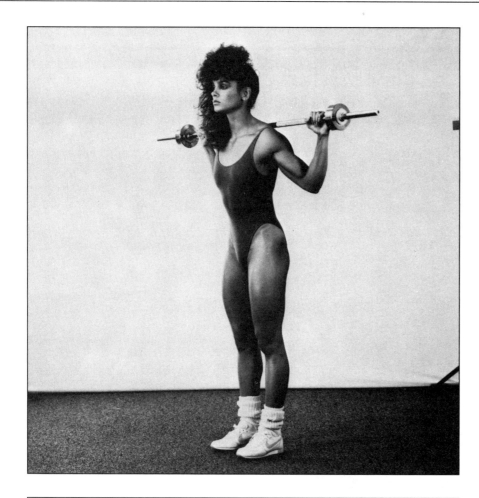

LUNGE (START)

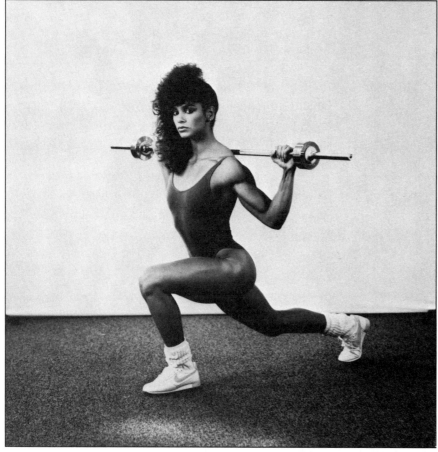

LUNGE (FINISH)

ONE-LEG TOE RAISE

This exercise develops the calf muscles.

DIRECTIONS	• With a relatively heavy dumbbell in your right hand, stand on a block of wood about 6–8 inches high. • Place the ball of your right foot on the wooden block and let the heel and arch of your foot hang off the wood. • Keep your other foot off the block of wood and out of the way. (You may use your left arm to hold on to something in order to keep balance.)
MOVEMENT	• Slowly let your right heel descend toward the floor, as low as possible, getting a full stretch in the calf muscle. • Slowly ascend to starting position and repeat this movement until you have performed the correct number of repetitions for your set. • Repeat the movement for your left leg. • Be sure to do three full sets for *each* leg, alternating a full set for right, then a full set for left, and so on.
SUGGESTIONS	You may alter the position of your toes for each of the three sets. The first set, toes may be pointed straight ahead, the second set toes pointed outward, and the third set toes pointed inward. This ensures a complete calf development.
DON'TS	Do not shorten the length of the drop when lowering your heel. Go all the way down and feel that stretch.

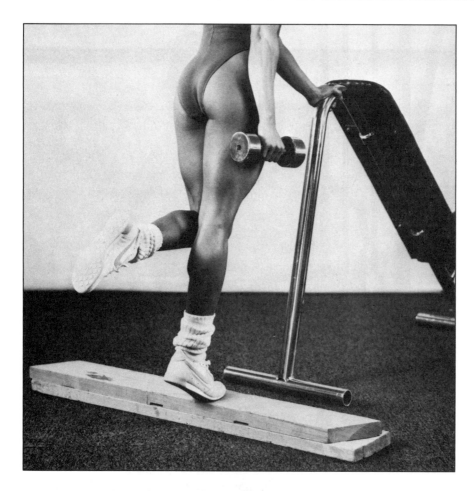

ONE-LEG TOE RAISE (START)

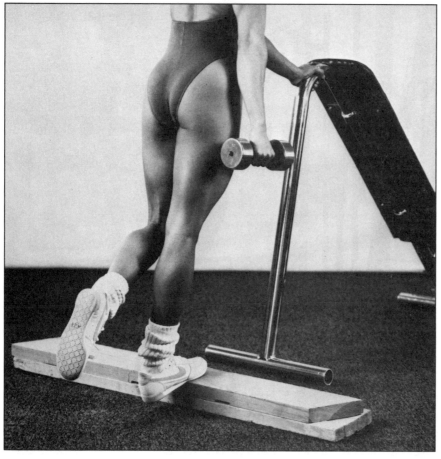

ONE-LEG TOE RAISE (FINISH)

SQUAT

This exercise develops the front quadriceps (thigh muscle). It also helps to firm the gluteus maximus (buttock muscle).

DIRECTIONS

- Place a barbell across your shoulders, behind your neck, and place your hands on the barbell in a comfortable position, balancing it on your trapezius muscles.

- Stand with your feet shoulder width apart. Tighten your abdomen and stand straight, look directly ahead of you, and focus on a point so that you can keep your head and back straight throughout the exercise.

MOVEMENT

- Slowly lower yourself into a squatting position by bending your legs at the knees. (As you are bending, be sure to keep your knees in direct line with your feet. That is, prevent the tendency of your knees to move out of line with your feet.)

- Descend as low as your knees will allow and slowly return to starting position. Repeat the movement until you have performed the correct number of repetitions for your set.

SUGGESTIONS

Many people prefer to do the squat with a two-by-four placed under the heels of their feet. This helps maintain balance. Vary the position of your toes. You may do the first set with toes pointed outward at the 45-degree angle, the second set with toes pointed straight ahead, and the third set with toes pointed completely outward.

DON'TS

Do not bounce when you reach the lowest point of the movement in an attempt to give yourself momentum to rise to starting position. Rather, use the strength of your quadriceps (thigh muscles) to elevate you. Continually picture the quadriceps taking the shape you have in mind when you look in the mirror and see your ideal body.

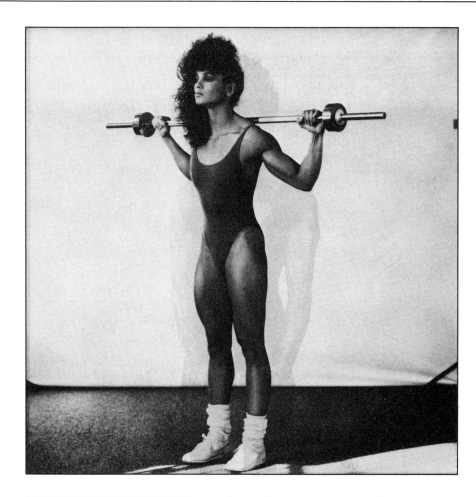

SQUAT (START)

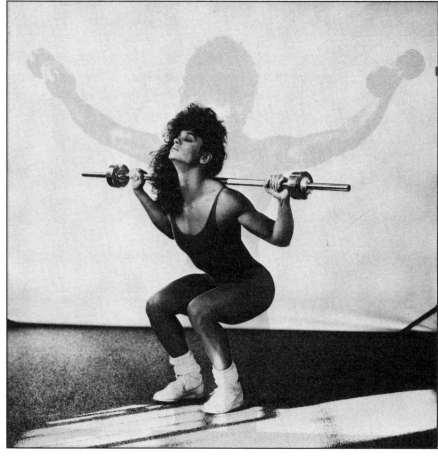

SQUAT (FINISH)

LEG EXTENSION

This exercise develops your front quadriceps (thigh muscles). It can be done on the Universal Gym, the Nautilus, or a freestanding machine.

DIRECTIONS

- Sit in the machine seat and place your insteps under the roller pads.

- Hold on to the handles or the side of the seat on either side of you.

MOVEMENT

- Slowly raise your legs until they are straight out in front of you and hold that position for one second.

- Slowly return to starting position and repeat the movement until you have performed the correct number of repetitions for your set.

SUGGESTIONS

As you perform the movement, watch your quadriceps contract and expand and visualize the definition that is being formed.

DON'TS

Do not bounce the weight up and let it drop down in an attempt to make the exercise easier by building up momentum. You must continually control the weight, moving slowly up and down. Flex your quadriceps. Concentrate.

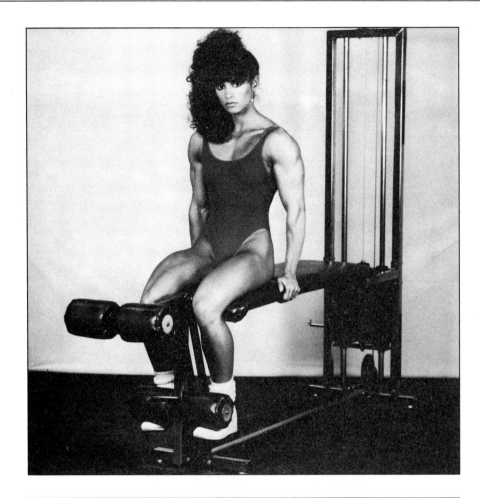

LEG EXTENSION (START)

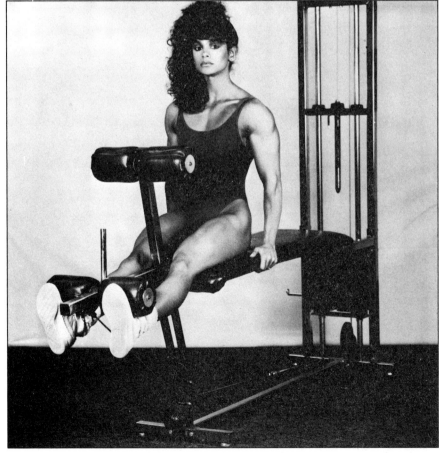

LEG EXTENSION (FINISH)

LEG CURL

This exercise develops the muscle of the back thigh, the biceps femoris (hamstring muscle). It can be performed on the Universal Gym, the Nautilus, or a freestanding machine.

DIRECTIONS

- Lie on the padded bench of the machine, face down, with your knees just touching the lower edge of the bench.

- Place the heels of your feet under the roller pads and hold on to the handles or the bench on either side of you.

MOVEMENT

- Slowly bend your legs at the knee, raising your feet upward until your legs are perpendicular to the floor.

- Hold the position for a split second and slowly return to starting position.

- Repeat the movement until you have performed the correct number of repetitions for your set.

SUGGESTIONS

Concentrate on your hamstring muscles as you do the exercise. Be sure to tighten the muscles, flexing as hard as possible as you raise your legs.

DON'TS

Do not let your back hump up. Keep your abdomen flat on the bench. Do not swing the weight up and do not drop it down. Control the weight at all times as you slowly lower and raise it.

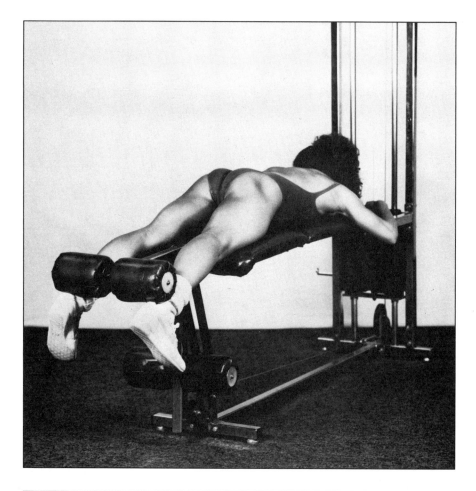

LEG CURL (START)

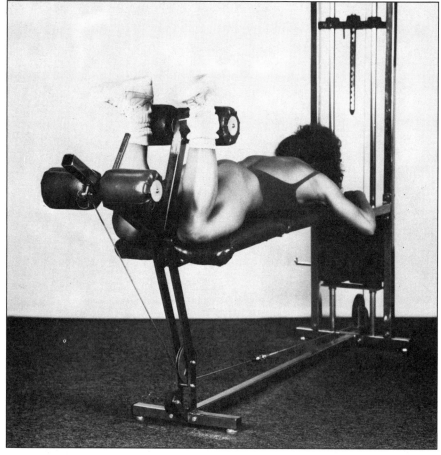

LEG CURL (FINISH)

ABDOMINAL ROUTINE

The abdominals require a different workout than do other body parts. They are not trained with weights, except for optional light weights on occasion, and then the weight remains constant for each set.

Abdominals must be treated with more repetitions than other body parts. Start out with 15 repetitions per set for each exercise and eventually work up to a minimum of 25 repetitions per set. Your eventual goal will be to go as high as 50 repetitions for each of your abdominal sets. This may take you a year, and that is fine.

Do not try to add too many repetitions to your set of 15 at one time. One additional rep every time you work out is sufficient.

In order to achieve hard, shapely muscles in your stomach area, and to get rid of unsightly fat, you must hit your abdominal area hard and keep on hitting it. Notice that the abdominals are the only muscle group that we ask you to work every workout day. Notice also that we give you more exercises for your abdominals than for any other body part.

INCLINE BENCH LEG RAISE

This exercise develops the lower abdominal muscles.

DIRECTIONS

- Place a 12-inch block of wood or other object under an exercise bench so that the bench is on a 45-degree incline. (You may use a regular sit-up board that can be adjusted to a moderate-to-steep angle, or you may use an incline bench.)

- Lie on the bench with your calves touching the end of the bench and your hands placed under your upper thighs or buttocks. Keep your head raised rather than relaxed.

MOVEMENT

- Slowly raise your legs until they are perpendicular to your body and slowly return to starting position. Without resting for a split second, repeat the movement until you have completed the correct number of repetitions for your set.

SUGGESTIONS

When you have completed your last set, try holding your legs 3 inches off the bench for 10 seconds. While doing this, flex (tighten, squeeze) your lower and upper abdominals. This helps tighten the abdominals.

DON'TS

Do not swing your legs up into the air or let your legs drop down, but raise them and lower them slowly, with control. Be careful not to bend your knees. Keep your legs straight at all times. Concentrate.

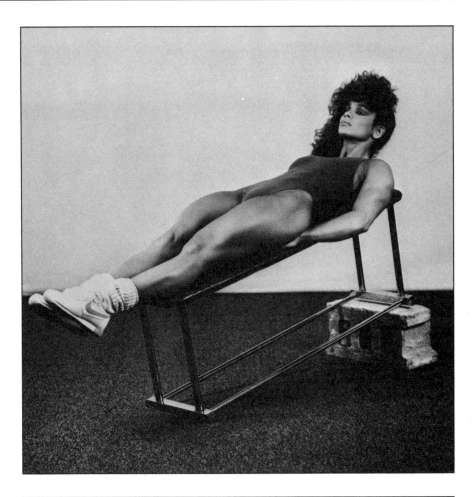

INCLINE BENCH LEG RAISE
(START)

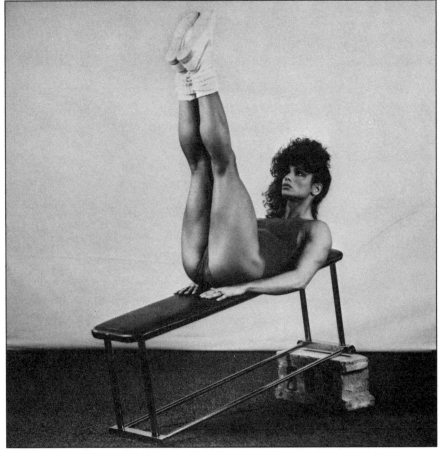

INCLINE BENCH LEG RAISE
(FINISH)

STRAIGHT BENCH SIT-UP

This exercise develops the upper half of your abdominals.

DIRECTIONS

- Lie flat on your back on a padded sit-up board, placing your feet under the leather strap or roller pads.

- Bend your knees slightly and cross your arms in front of you, fingertips touching your shoulders.

MOVEMENT

- Slowly rise, curling yourself upward until you are perpendicular to the floor.

- Without hesitation slowly return to starting position and immediately repeat the movement until you have completed the correct number of repetitions for your set.

SUGGESTIONS

Abdominal muscles need more stress than other muscles. Therefore you must add 5 repetitions each week (to your beginning 15) until you have reached 40 and are able to do 3 sets of 40. If you are ambitious, you may go as high as 3 sets of 50. You may also want to vary the exercise by twisting your body as you go up. In this case, place your hands behind your neck and alternately touch your right elbow to your left knee and your left elbow to your right knee.

DON'TS

Do not bounce off the board or bench. Slowly raise and lower yourself as you tighten your abdominal muscles.

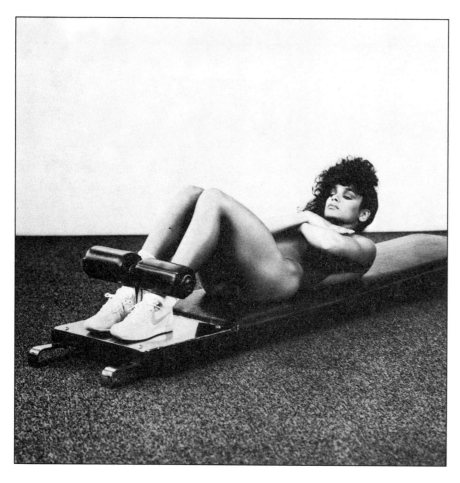

STRAIGHT BENCH SIT-UP (START)

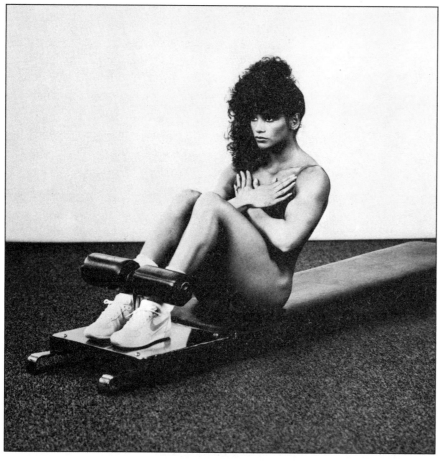

STRAIGHT BENCH SIT-UP (FINISH)

ROMAN CHAIR SIT-UP WITH A WEIGHT

This exercise develops the muscles of the entire abdominal area (lower and upper).

DIRECTIONS

- With a light weight in your hands, seat yourself in the Roman chair or hyperextension bench, placing your feet under the foot holder.

- Place the weight in the center of your body (it should cross your chest, abdomen, waist area) and hold it with both hands (your hands should be crossed over the weight in front of you).

- Sit up so that your body is perpendicular to the floor.

MOVEMENT

- Slowly lower your body until you are almost parallel to the floor, flexing (squeezing) your abdominal muscles at all times.

- Continuing to flex your abdominal muscles, slowly return to starting position and repeat the movement until you have completed the correct number of repetitions for your set.

SUGGESTIONS

Wrap the weight in a towel so that the natural dye does not rub off on your clothing. After two weeks graduate to 15 pounds, and in another two weeks, 20 pounds. If you are ambitious you may go as high as 25 pounds. You need not increase your repetitions, but you may if you wish to see more rapid development of the abdominals. In this case you may work your way up to 25, adding 2 repetitions per week. Do not use heavy weights if you have back problems.

DON'TS

Do not let your body drop down. Control the movement at all times. Concentrate on the muscles being worked.

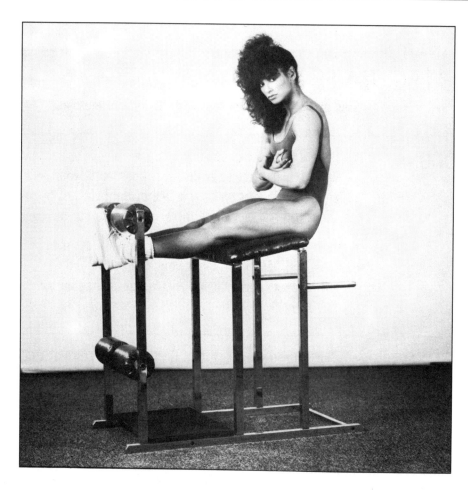

ROMAN CHAIR SIT-UP
WITH A WEIGHT (START)

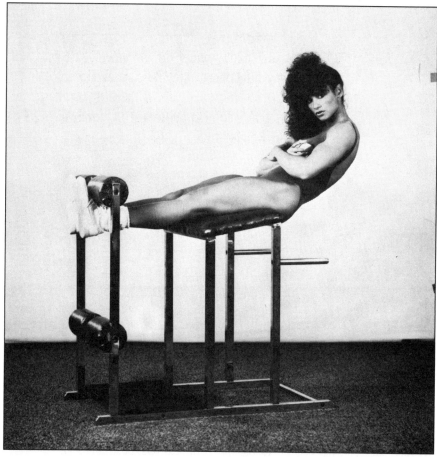

ROMAN CHAIR SIT-UP
WITH A WEIGHT (FINISH)

BENCH LEG RAISE WITH A WEIGHT

This exercise develops the lower abdominal muscles.

DIRECTIONS	• Place a 3- or a 5-pound weight between your ankles and lie on a flat exercise bench or a floorboard, your back and your hips flat on the surface of the bench or board. (Your legs will only touch the bench or board at the heel.)
	• Hold on to the bench or board on either side, near your hips, and bend your knees very slightly. (If you wish, you may lie on your hands instead of holding on to the bench.)
MOVEMENT	• Slowly raise your legs until they are perpendicular to the floor and slowly lower them to starting position.
	• Repeat the movement immediately, until you have completed the correct number of repetitions for your set.
SUGGESTIONS	Flex (tighten and squeeze) your lower abdominal muscles throughout the exercise.
DON'TS	Do not let your mind wander for a moment: you could let go of the weight! Concentrate. Be careful. Do not use a weight that is too heavy for you. If there is any danger of your not being able to hold the weight between your feet, use a lighter weight.

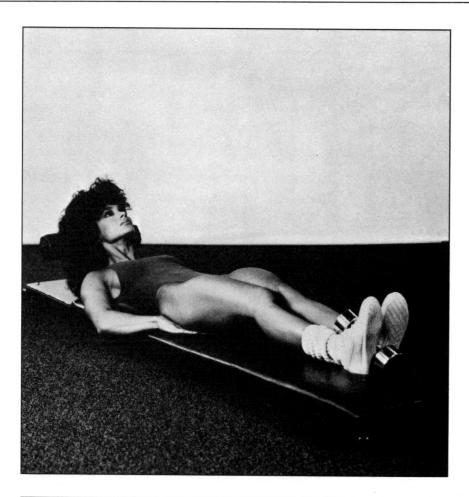

BENCH LEG RAISE WITH A WEIGHT
(START)

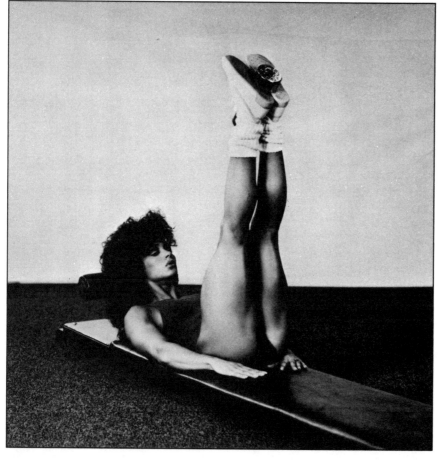

BENCH LEG RAISE WITH A WEIGHT
(FINISH)

SERRATUS PULL

This exercise develops your anterior serratus (side abdominal) muscles. (See anatomy chart, pp. 12–13.)

DIRECTIONS

- Grip the handle of the floor Universal Gym or of the free-standing machine pulley in your right hand, standing sideways to the machine.

- Bend toward the machine, stretching your left side slightly. You should feel the weight of the machine on your right hand. You are now in starting position.

MOVEMENT

- Slowly bend to your left side, crunching your waist on your left side and stretching your waist at your right side. (Be sure to feel the stretch and crunch on your right and left sides. Do not do the work with your arm.)

- Bend until your fingertips reach about thigh level, and slowly return to starting position.

- Repeat the movement until you have performed the correct number of repetitions for your set.

- Repeat the set for your left side.

SUGGESTIONS

You may wish to do this exercise using an overhead pulley (see photo p. 128). In this case you may use the lateral machine and make a triangle with your right arm, bending it at the elbow and keeping your left arm from doing the work, crunching only at the waist.

DON'TS

Do not do the work with your arms. Use your free arm from time to time to feel your working side to be sure that the muscles in your serratus area (side) are "working."

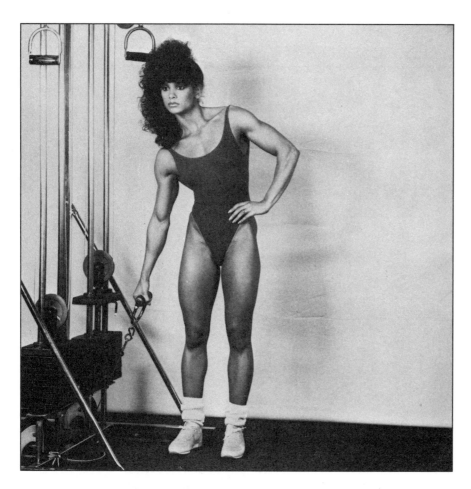

SERRATUS PULL (START)

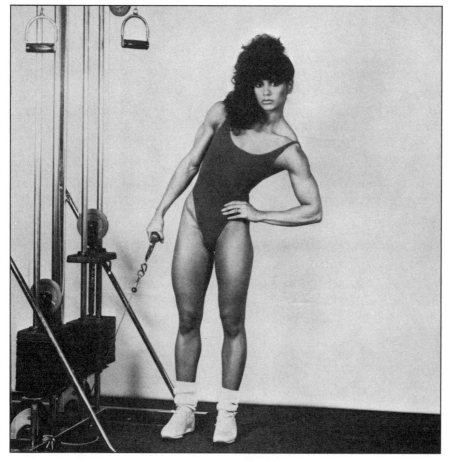

SERRATUS PULL (FINISH)

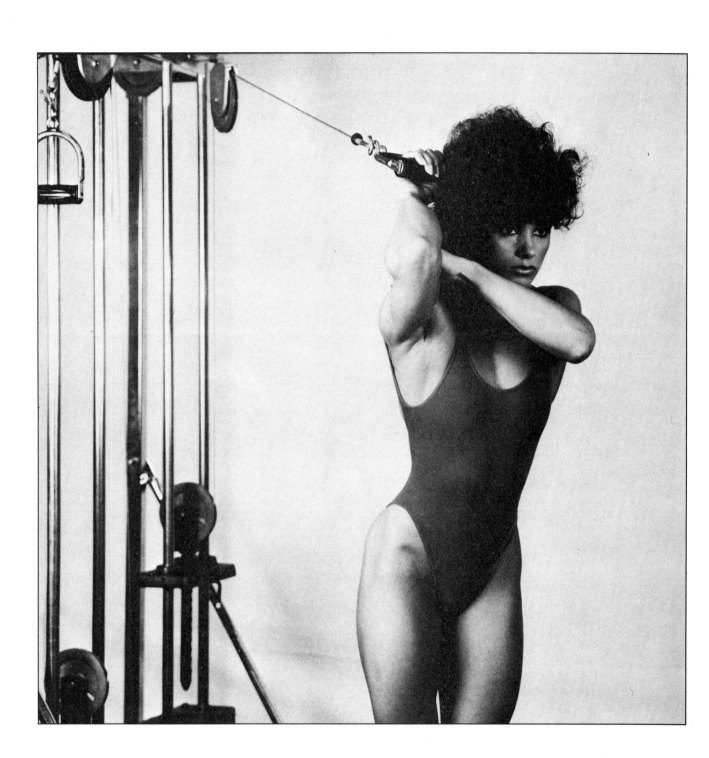

THE SLIM BODY WORKOUT

Muscles increase in mass and density when they are progressively forced to do more work. If you are too thin, you will want to increase your size or change your shape without increasing fat (which is unshapely). By following the program especially created for slim bodies, you will develop shapely muscles and burn off excess body fat. It is possible to be "fat" and underweight. If your body composition is 35 percent fat (it should never be more than 20–25 percent fat), then you are fat even though you may be underweight according to the chart.

Careful diet (explained in Chapter Ten) and intelligent workouts will help you form the perfectly symmetrical, shapely body that is your goal.

As a slim body, the principle of heavy versus light is important to you. The workouts described here require you to perform three sets per exercise. For each set, you will select a beginning weight that enables you to do 10 repetitions for the first set with some struggle. You will raise the weight for the second set so that you can get only 8 repetitions with a struggle. For the third set you will raise the weight so that 6 repetitions are difficult. By raising the weight and keeping it heavy, you are helping your body to build needed mass which will give you the shapely form you desire.

The principle behind the Hard Bodies slim body workout involves heavy weights and low repetitions. This method brings about the maximum building of muscle or body mass. Since a woman who is too slim does not want to gain fat when she gains weight, we ask her to work her muscles a bit harder than others. A thin woman who wants to be more shapely must work out with heavier weights in order to build shapely muscles and to place them exactly where she wants them (on her skinny legs, or her flat buttocks, on her too-thin arms, on her bony shoulders, etc.).

By using heavy weights and low repetitions, the muscles are forced to grow. They are doing hard work and at the same time are given time to rest and recuperate for the next set, which challenges them to grow even more.

BEGINNING THE WORKOUT

- Do 3 sets of 6–10 repetitions for each exercise, starting with light weight on the first set and adding more weight in each successive set.
- There are 3 exercises for each body part except legs (for which there are 4) and abdominals (for which there are 5).
- There are 9 sets for each body part except legs (12) and abdominals (15).
- You will do chest, shoulders, back, and abdominals on one training day.
- You will do biceps, triceps, legs, and abdominals on the next training day.
- You will train 4 days a week, working each part of the body twice a week, except for the abdominals, which you will work four days a week.

HOW TO DETERMINE YOUR BEGINNING WEIGHT

Each exercise will involve different equipment (dumbbells, barbells, machines, etc.), will stress different muscles, and will require the use of different weights. Determine your beginning weight by the following method:

- Select a weight which is heavy enough to make it a challenge to get 10 repetitions but not so heavy that you have to strain or do the exercise incorrectly.
- Perform 10 repetitions with that weight.
- Add 2–10 pounds to that weight and perform at least 8 repetitions for your

second set. (If you got 10 repetitions with the lighter weight, you should be able to get 8 repetitions with a slightly heavier weight.)
- Add 2–10 pounds to that weight and perform at least 6 repetitions for your third set.
- When you have completed 3 sets of one exercise, move to the next exercise.

PERFORMING THE EXERCISES

Do each exercise in the following manner: Do 3 sets of each exercise. Do the first set at 10 repetitions, the second at 8 repetitions, and the third at 6 repetitions. For each set you must raise the weight. Remember, after a week or two the starting weight should become too easy and you should begin with more weight. For example:

CHEST ROUTINE

Bench Press:	Set 1.	50 pounds, 10 repetitions
	Set 2.	60 pounds, 8 repetitions
	Set 3.	70 pounds, 6 repetitions
Incline Flye:	Set 1.	10 pounds, 10 repetitions
	Set 2.	15 pounds, 8 repetitions
	Set 3.	20 pounds, 6 repetitions
Cross Bench Pullovers:	Set 1.	20 pounds, 10 repetitions
	Set 2.	25 pounds, 8 repetitions
	Set 3.	30 pounds, 6 repetitions

And so on.

RAISING THE BEGINNING WEIGHT IN A WEEK OR TWO

After a few weeks you will notice that your beginning weight will be too easy. Using the above example of the bench press, after a few weeks (maybe sooner, maybe a lot longer—even two months but that is unlikely) the beginning weight of 50 pounds is so easy that the weight seems to fly up as you push it, and you know you could really get more than 10 repetitions. This is a sign that it is time to change the weight. Clearly, if it is obvious to you that you could get more than 10 repetitions without any trouble, it is time to raise your beginning weight. Raise your beginning weight to 60 pounds. Now your second set will be 70 at 8 reps and your final set will be 80 at 6 reps. Continue to raise your beginning weight whenever the need arises. In a year's time you will be surprised at the difference. One of our clients started out at 30 pounds for her beginning weight and a year later was beginning with 100 pounds.

Always keep in mind, you have to push yourself. It is necessary to work hard for muscles, but it is well worth it in the long run. The time and energy are a permanent investment in a beautiful, youthful, sensual body. Your goal should be to work as hard as you can each workout day.

RESTING

You can rest as long as 60 seconds between sets, but 30 seconds should be quite enough. Since you are lifting heavy weights, your muscles will probably need at least a 30-second rest. If you find that you don't need any rest at all, chances are you are not challenging your muscles enough and your weights are too light.

AEROBIC REQUIREMENT

Although you are not overweight, we want you to do some aerobics for skin tone and overall fitness (heart and lung capacity). Spend 20 minutes, three times a week, either riding a stationary bicycle, running, jumping rope, or swimming. You may fit these three 20-minute sessions into any time slot of any day you wish. Just be sure to get them in.

FINE-TUNING

If you have misproportioned areas such as big legs and a thin upper body, or a bulging stomach—or if you want results more quickly—turn to Chapter Nine and follow the instructions for attacking the troublesome body parts. This will involve you in some extra exercises, including floor exercises. You do not have to begin working on troublesome body parts immediately, however. You may wait two or three months, or you may choose to continue your slim body workout for six months and then zero in on the problem areas. Your slim body workout is designed to hit at your troublesome parts anyway.

BREAKING IN

Complete only 1 set of each exercise for the first training day. For example, instead of 3 sets of the incline bench press, do 1 set and move to the next exercise, incline flyes. Perform one set of that exercise and move to the next exercise, the cross bench pullover.

Follow the same breaking-in light workout on your second training day, when you do biceps, triceps, and legs. You will be doing only 1 set of repetitions per exercise instead of 3.

Continue doing only 1 set per exercise for the first training week. You will have trained four times that first week, twice for each body part except abdominals, which you will have trained four times.

By your second week you are ready to do 2 sets per exercise. Do the 2 sets for each exercise for each of the four training days that week.

By your third week you are ready to do your full workout of 3 sets per exercise. Now you can follow the prescribed instructions exactly. Your muscles will have been broken in gently and the soreness will have been bearable.

Some ambitious women want to start out with all three sets per exercise the first day. Don't. It results in undue soreness and a temptation to quit. You will feel the effects even starting slowly.

The full routine should take 90 minutes.

CHEST ROUTINE

DECLINE BENCH PRESS

This exercise develops the entire pectoral (breast) area.

DIRECTIONS	• Lie on a decline bench (you may place a block of wood or other object under the foot of the bench to produce a decline) holding a barbell with your hands shoulder width apart. • Raise the barbell until your arms are fully extended. (The barbell should be held just above your breast area.)
MOVEMENT	• Slowly lower the barbell until it just grazes your breast area and immediately raise it to starting position. • Without pausing, repeat the movement until you have completed the correct number of repetitions for your set.
SUGGESTIONS	Vary the grip from time to time. You may grip the barbell with your hands 10 inches apart, 12 inches apart, and so on.
DON'TS	Do not let the bar drop on the downward movement. Control it at all times. Concentrate on the pectoral area as you perform the movement. Flex your chest as you lift the bar and let it stretch out as you lower the bar. Never rest between repetitions.
INCLINE FLYE	Follow the exercise description on p. 70.
CROSS BENCH PULLOVER	Follow the exercise description on p. 72.

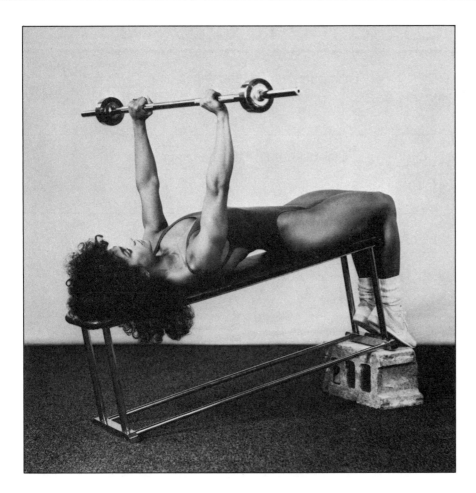

DECLINE BENCH PRESS (START)

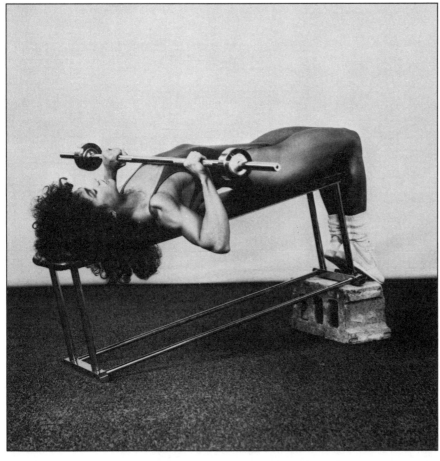

DECLINE BENCH PRESS (FINISH)

SHOULDER ROUTINE

MILITARY PRESS TO THE FRONT	Follow the exercise description on p. 76.
SIDE LATERAL RAISE	Follow the exercise description on p. 78.
UPRIGHT ROW	Follow the exercise description on p. 80.

BACK ROUTINE

SEATED PULLEY ROW	Follow the exercise description on p. 84.
DUMBBELL BENT ROW	Follow the exercise description on p. 86.
LAT MACHINE PULLDOWN TO THE FRONT	Follow the exercise description on p. 88.

BICEPS ROUTINE

STANDING BARBELL CURL	Follow the exercise description on p. 92.
ONE-ARM PREACHER CURL	Follow the exercise description on p. 94.
PULLEY CURL	Follow the exercise description on p. 96.

T R I C E P S   R O U T I N E

DUMBBELL KICKBACK

This exercise develops the entire triceps area.

DIRECTIONS	• Hold a dumbbell in your left hand and lean against an exercise bench with your right hand and knee, bending at the waist so that your back is parallel to the floor. • Keeping your left upper arm pinned to your side, let your left forearm (from elbow to hand) drop down in a perpendicular line with the floor. (The dumbbell is held with palm toward the body.)
MOVEMENT	• Slowly straighten your arm toward your rear, using the elbow as a hinge. • Slowly return the weight to starting position and repeat the movement until you have completed the correct number of repetitions for your set. • Repeat the exercise for your right arm and repeat with left and right arms until you have completed 3 sets.
SUGGESTIONS	It is necessary to use a light weight for this exercise and to do it in a strict fashion. Flex your triceps and visualize the muscle as you perform the exercise.
DON'TS	Do not let your elbow wander away (outwards) from your waist.
ONE-ARM DUMBBELL TRICEPS EXTENSION	Follow the exercise description on p. 102.
PULLEY PUSHDOWN	Follow the exercise description on p. 104.

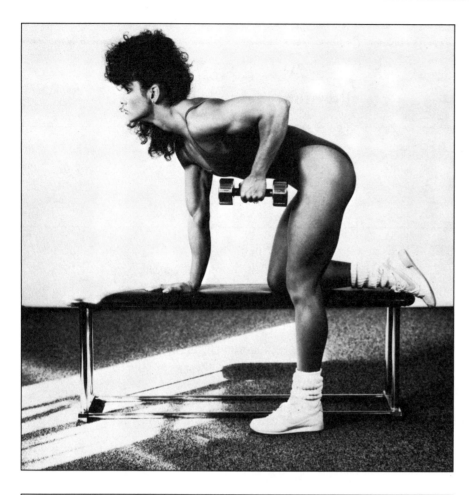

DUMBBELL KICKBACK (START)

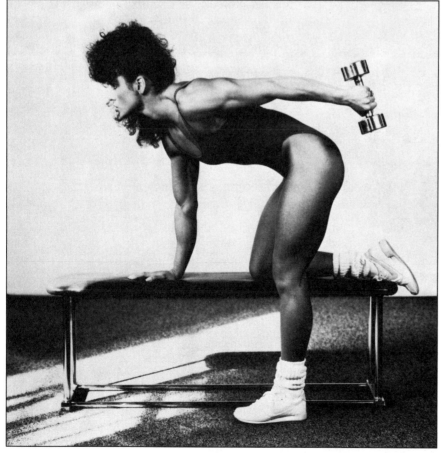

DUMBBELL KICKBACK (FINISH)

LEG ROUTINE

DONKEY CALF RAISE

This exercise develops your calf muscles.

DIRECTIONS	• Stand on a thick block of wood with the balls of your feet on the wood and your heels off the wood. • Lean over an incline bench.
MOVEMENT	• Lower your heels to the lowest possible point and then slowly raise them, standing as high on your toes as possible. • Slowly lower yourself to starting position. • Repeat this movement until you have performed the correct number of repetitions for your set.
SUGGESTIONS	You may wear a special belt around your waist with a weight attached. This provides additional weight and causes your calf muscles to work harder. You may alter the position of your toes from time to time, placing them straight ahead, pointed outward, and pointed inward. This ensures even development of the calf muscles.
SQUAT	Follow the exercise description on p. 110.
LEG EXTENSION	Follow the exercise description on p. 112.
LEG CURL	Follow the exercise description on p. 114.

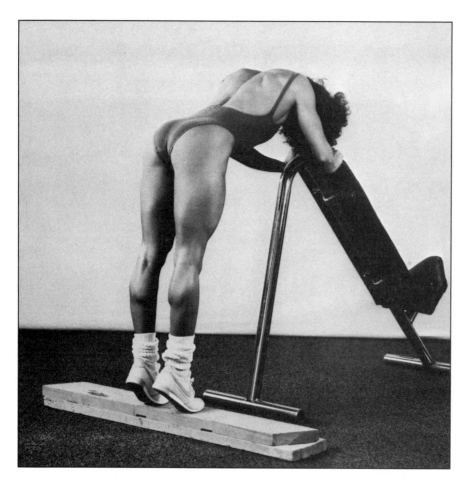

DONKEY CALF RAISE (START)

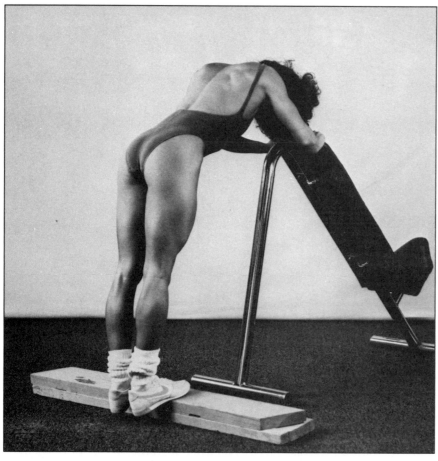

DONKEY CALF RAISE (FINISH)

ABDOMINAL ROUTINE

The abdominals are treated differently than other body parts. They are not usually trained with weights, except for optional light weights on occasion, and then the weight remains constant for each set.

For this reason, the abdominals require more repetitions than other body parts. Start out each set with 15 repetitions and eventually work up to a minimum of 25 repetitions per set. Your eventual goal will be to go as high as 50 repetitions per set of every abdominal exercise. This can take up to a year, and that's fine.

Do not add too many repetitions to your starting 15 at one session. Simply add a rep or two each time you work out. You can stay at the same number of reps for a while before increasing them. But remember, the goal is tight abdominals with no excess body fat, and to achieve this goal you must work that area hard.

Even though you are slim, body fat deposits itself on your abdomen, so you must hit that area harder than any other. Notice that the abdominals are the only muscle group that we ask you to exercise every workout day.

CRUNCH

This exercise develops the upper abdominals.

DIRECTIONS	• Lie flat on your back, on the floor, with your legs over a flat exercise bench. There should be a 90-degree bend at the waist. • Fold your hands behind your neck.
MOVEMENT	• Slowly lift yourself up, using only your shoulders and lower abdominal muscles in unison. • Rise only high enough to lift your entire shoulder area off the floor. Do not go higher. • Slowly lower yourself to starting position and repeat the movement until you have performed the correct number of repetitions for your set.
SUGGESTIONS	Add 1 repetition to your original 15 each time you work out (4 repetitions a week) until you have reached 30 repetitions. You may stop there, but if you wish, you may go as high as 50 repetitions.
DON'TS	Do not jerk yourself off the floor. Slowly rise to the upper position and then, in total control, slowly lower yourself. Remember to flex your abdominal muscles at all times.
STRAIGHT BENCH SIT-UP	Follow the exercise description on p. 120.
ROMAN CHAIR SIT-UP WITH A WEIGHT	Follow the exercise description on p. 122.
BENCH LEG RAISE WITH A WEIGHT	Follow the exercise description on p. 124.
SERRATUS PULL	Follow the exercise description on p. 126.

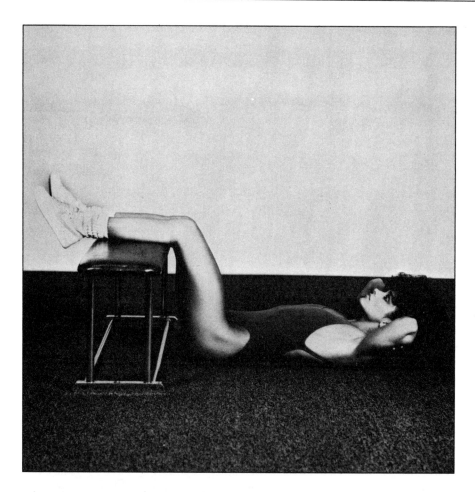

CRUNCH (START)

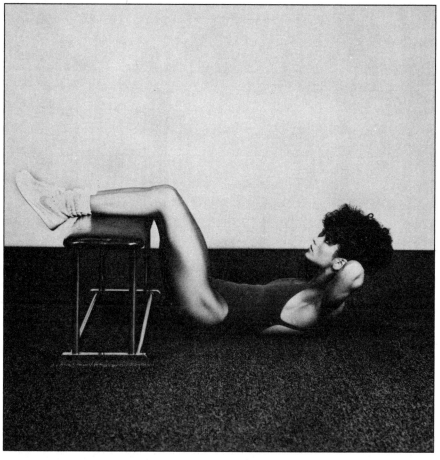

CRUNCH (FINISH)

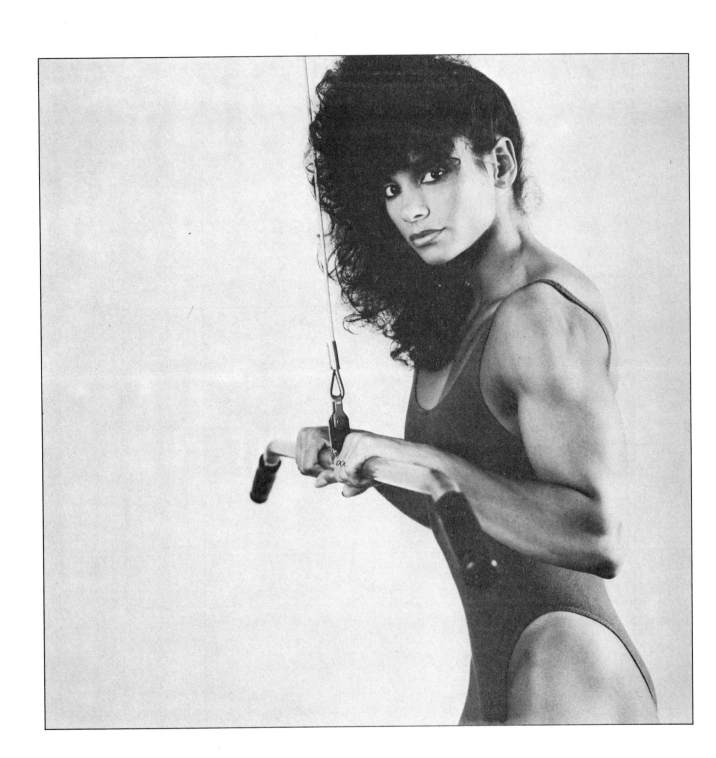

THE BULKY BODY WORKOUT

Women who are oversized are carrying too much body mass. Their problem is that of reduction, not of muscle but of fat and water. It is physically impossible to lose more than two to two and a half pounds a week of body fat. Those who claim to have lost more weight than that, have lost water and even muscle. For this reason the realistic diet plan explained in Chapter Ten is especially important with our specialized workout for the bulky body.

Many women who are already bigger than they want to be fear that by working out with weights they will become too muscular and appear even bigger. This will not happen. It is a myth which must quickly be dispelled with facts.

Fat takes up a lot more space than muscle. With our special program, bulky bodies will reduce body fat and at the same time put on muscle. While muscle weighs more than fat, it takes up *much less* space. For example, think of the fat surrounding a piece of steak and compare it to the meat or "muscle" of the steak. A two-inch-square piece of fat will weigh much less on a food-measuring scale than a two-inch-square piece of lean meat. Try it.

As soon as you begin to work out, there will be a noticeable change in your body composition. Clothing will begin to fit more loosely before there is any weight loss. People will begin to comment on how much weight you seem to be losing, but what is actually happening is the loss of large amounts of body fat and the addition of small amounts of muscle. (It takes a long time to put on solid muscle, but once the muscle is there it remains as a permanent body shaper as long as you maintain a reasonable workout schedule.)

The principle behind the Hard Bodies bulky body workout is low weights and high repetitions. This combination brings about the maximum burning of fat along with the building of shapely muscles. When muscles are worked at a steady pace, without prolonged rest, they are forced to grow stronger and denser (more shapely), and calories are burned more efficiently. By not allowing the body to rest too long, you produce an aerobic effect. The idea is to sustain a heartbeat that is accelerated for more than twenty minutes; if you follow our routine, gradually decreasing your rest periods, this aerobic effect will be achieved.

BEGINNING THE WORKOUT

- Do three sets of 12–15 repetitions for each exercise.
- There are 5 exercises for each body part with the exception of legs (for which there are 6) and abdominals (for which there are 7).
- There are 15 sets for each body part, except for legs (18) and abdominals (21).
- You will do chest, shoulders, back, and abdominals on one training day.
- You will do biceps, triceps, legs, and abdominals on the next training day.
- You will train 4 days per week, working each part of the body twice a week, except for the abdominals, which you will work 4 times a week.

HOW TO DETERMINE YOUR BEGINNING WEIGHT

Each exercise will involve different equipment (dumbbells, barbells, machines), will stress different muscles, and will require various weights. Determine your beginning weight by the following method:

- Select a light weight.
- Perform 15 repetitions with that weight.
- Add 2–10 pounds to that weight and perform another 15 repetitions. (If you

can get only 12 repetitions, keep that weight. Do not go higher. If you can get 15 repetitions, select another weight 2–10 pounds higher for your third set.)

• Perform your third set with 12–15 repetitions.

The idea is to try to make your muscles work harder and maintain 12–15 repetitions. You want to keep the repetitions high in order to burn fat at the fastest possible rate, and to build small, dense muscles.

Now that you have completed 3 sets of one exercise you are ready to move on to the next exercise.

In doing the bench press, for example, if you do the first set at 30 pounds, 15 repetitions, your next set will be 40 pounds. If you get only 12 repetitions, remain at that weight for the third and final set (of 12 reps).

PERFORMING THE EXERCISES

Do 3 sets of each exercise, and do 12–15 repetitions for each set. Go as fast as you can, allowing yourself as little rest as possible consistent with doing the exercise in perfectly strict form. This is important. The form must *never* be sacrificed for speed. Rest for 15–45 seconds whenever you need to. Samples:

CHEST ROUTINE

Pec Deck Flye:	Set 1.	40 pounds, 15 repetitions
	Set 2.	40 pounds, 12 repetitions
	Set 3.	40 pounds, 12 repetitions
Flat Bench Press:	Set 1.	40 pounds, 15 repetitions
	Set 2.	40 pounds, 15 repetitions
	Set 3.	40 pounds, 15 repetitions
Incline Flye:	Set 1.	15 pounds, 15 repetitions
	Set 2.	15 pounds, 12 repetitions
	Set 3.	15 pounds, 12 repetitions
Cross Bench Pullover:	Set 1.	15 pounds, 15 repetitions
	Set 2.	15 pounds, 15 repetitions
	Set 3.	15 pounds, 12 repetitions

Cable Crossover: Set 1. 7½ pounds, 15 repetitions
                  Set 2. 7½ pounds, 12 repetitions
                  Set 3. 7½ pounds, 12 repetitions

And so on.

RAISING THE BEGINNING WEIGHT IN A WEEK OR TWO

After a few weeks you will notice that working with your beginning weight has become too easy. Using the example of the bench press, after a few weeks (maybe sooner) the beginning weight of 40 pounds will be so easy that the weight seems to fly up when you push it. It will become obvious that you are not "working" hard enough. Increase your beginning weight to 50 pounds and try to increase your second set to 60 pounds and get at least 12 repetitions. If you cannot, just keep all three sets at 50 pounds until you can increase the beginning weight to 60 pounds (probably in a few more weeks).

Usually, if you can get 15 repetitions with a given weight, you can get 12 repetitions with a slightly higher weight. Push yourself a little. Remember: no pain, no gain. The harder you work, the harder your body will be. No hard work, no hard body.

RESTING

Rest 15–45 seconds between each set. But remember, the faster you go (without rushing and doing incomplete repetitions), the more fat you will burn.

AEROBIC REQUIREMENT

In addition to doing your bulky body workout, you must find four half-hour spaces to perform an aerobics exercise. You may run, ride a stationary bicycle, jump rope, or swim, but it must be for one half hour. Of course you may work up to it, beginning with 5 minutes and taking a few weeks to reach the half hour (add 5 minutes a week). This will help tone your skin and burn fat and at the same time condition your heart and lungs.

FINE-TUNING

At some point, probably after 2 months, you will want to turn to Chapter Nine and follow the instructions for zeroing in on troublesome body parts (such as sagging triceps or flabby thighs). This will involve you in some extra workouts, including floor exercises. You may choose to wait another four months before doing the extra work required to fine-tune your body. This is fine because your bulky body workout will be hitting those trouble spots anyway. The fine-tuning for troublesome body parts is provided for those who want results more quickly.

BREAKING IN

Complete only 1 set of each exercise for the first training day. For example, instead of doing 3 sets of the pec deck flye, do one set and move to the flat bench press. Perform only 1 set and move to the incline flye. Do only 1 set of that and move to the cross bench pullover. Do only 1 set of that and move to your final chest exercise, the cable crossover. You will continue to do only 1 set of each exercise for each body part that first training day.

Follow the same breaking-in light workout on your second training day, when you work biceps, triceps, and legs—only 1 set of repetitions per exercise instead of three.

Continue doing only one set per exercise for the first training week. You will have trained four times that first week, twice for each body part except four times for abdominals.

By your second week you are ready to do 2 sets per exercise. Complete 2 sets for each exercise each of the four training days that week.

By the third week you can do your full workout of 3 sets per exercise. Now you can follow the above instructions exactly. Your muscles will have been broken in gently and the soreness will be bearable.

Some ambitious women want to start out with the full program. Don't. It results in undue soreness and the temptation to quit. You will feel the effects even starting with 1 set per exercise.

The full routine should take 90 minutes.

CHEST ROUTINE

PEC DECK FLYE

This exercise develops the entire pectoral area. It can be done on the Nautilus or on a pec deck machine.

DIRECTIONS	• Sit in the machine seat after you have adjusted the seat so that your forearms fit comfortably behind the pads. • Place your forearms behind the pads and extend your arms outward as far toward your back as possible. (Your upper arms should be almost parallel to the floor throughout the exercise.)
MOVEMENT	• Slowly move your forearms toward each other until they are parallel, shoulder-width apart. • Slowly, controlling the weight, return to starting position and immediately repeat the movement until you have performed the correct number of repetitions for your set.
SUGGESTIONS	As you perform the exercise, concentrate on the contraction (the "in" movement) and the stretching (the "out" movement) of your pectoral (chest) area. Be sure to flex (squeeze) your chest muscles as you are pushing the pads in and to stretch your muscles fully as you are returning to starting position.
DON'TS	Do not lunge forward and jerk the pads in order to move them into position, and never allow the pads to pull you back to starting position. Control the weights at all times and remember to concentrate on the muscles being worked.
FLAT BENCH PRESS	Follow the exercise description on p. 66.
INCLINE FLYE	Follow the exercise description on p. 70.
CROSS BENCH PULLOVER	Follow the exercise description on p. 72.
CABLE CROSSOVER	Follow the exercise description on p. 68.

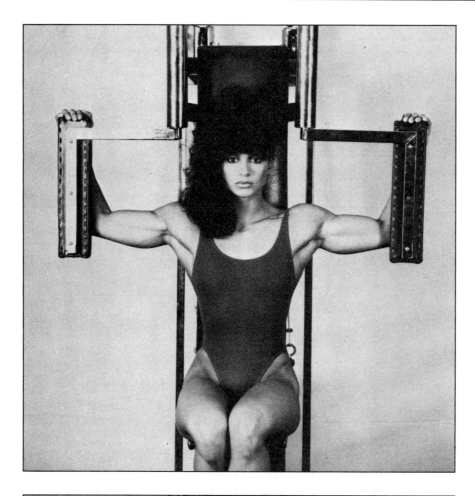

PEC DECK FLYE (START)

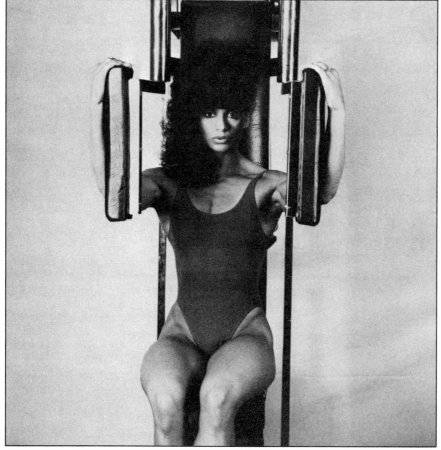

PEC DECK FLYE (FINISH)

S H O U L D E R   R O U T I N E

FRONT LATERAL RAISE

This exercise develops the front deltoid (front shoulder muscle; see anatomy chart, pp. 12–13).

DIRECTIONS	• With one dumbbell in each hand, stand with feet shoulder width apart and arms straight down in front of your thighs.
	• Holding the dumbbells with palms facing your body, flex your shoulders and prepare to begin the movement.
MOVEMENT	• Slowly raise your right arm, in front of your body, to shoulder height, and while you are slowly returning to starting position, raise your left arm to shoulder height.
	• While you are returning your left arm to starting position, raise your right arm to shoulder height, and so on, until you have completed the correct number of repetitions for your set with each arm.
SUGGESTIONS	It is possible to perform the exercise with a barbell, which would require you to raise and lower both arms at the same time. One might also use the two dumbbells in the same manner as a barbell, raising and lowering them both at the same time.
DON'TS	Do not allow your elbow to bend while performing the movement. Never swing your arm upward, but slowly raise it to shoulder height, controlling the weight at all times.
MILITARY PRESS TO THE FRONT	Follow the exercise description on p. 76.
SIDE LATERAL RAISE	Follow the exercise description on p. 78.
UPRIGHT ROW	Follow the exercise description on p. 80.
SIDE INCLINE LATERAL	Follow the exercise description on p. 74.

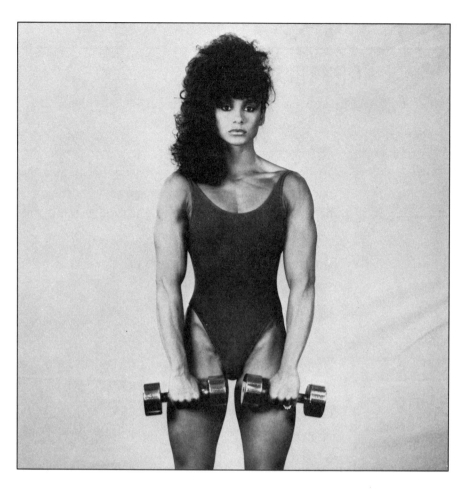

FRONT LATERAL RAISE
(START)

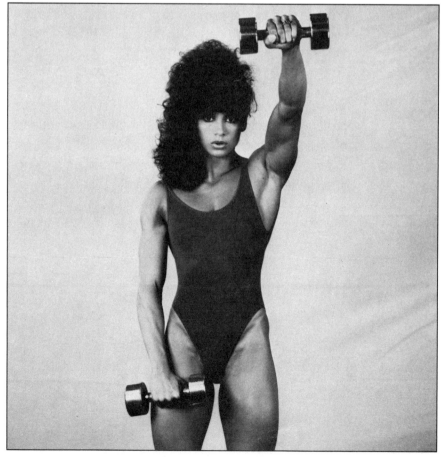

FRONT LATERAL RAISE
(FINISH)

BACK ROUTINE

HYPEREXTENSION

This exercise develops the lower back muscles, and provides a complete stretch for the back.

DIRECTIONS	• Get into position in the hyperextension bench by placing your heels under the padded bar and your abdomen over the larger padded surface, your waist touching the outer edge of the larger padded surface.
	• Bending at the waist, lean all the way down until you are perpendicular to the floor.
	• Clasp your hands behind your neck.
MOVEMENT	• Slowly raise your body until you are parallel to the floor (your back should be slightly arched).
	• Slowly lower yourself to starting position and repeat the movement until you have performed the correct number of repetitions for your set.
SUGGESTIONS	Some people hold a weight behind their head when they do this exercise. We do not recommend it because of the high risk of lower back and neck strain.
DON'TS	Do not jerk your body up and let it drop down to starting position. Control the movement at all times, concentrating on your lower back muscles. Flex (squeeze and tighten) your lower back muscles as you raise yourself up and let them stretch out as you lower yourself.

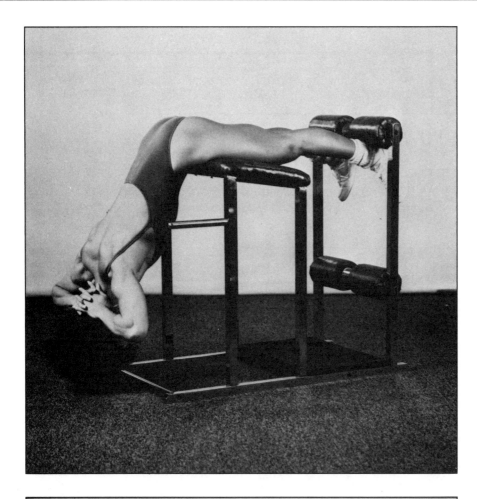

**HYPEREXTENSION
(START)**

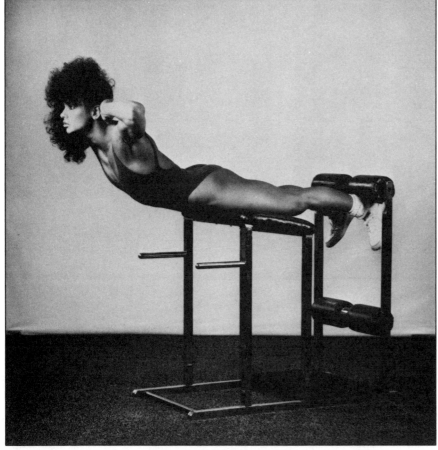

**HYPEREXTENSION
(FINISH)**

SEATED PULLEY ROW	Follow the exercise description on p. 84.
DUMBBELL BENT ROW	Follow the exercise description on p. 86.
LAT MACHINE PULLDOWN TO THE FRONT	Follow the exercise description on p. 88.
LAT MACHINE PULLDOWN TO THE BACK	Follow the exercise description on p. 88. Instead of pulling the bar down to touch your upper chest, lean forward and pull the bar down to touch the back of your neck and your trapezius muscles.

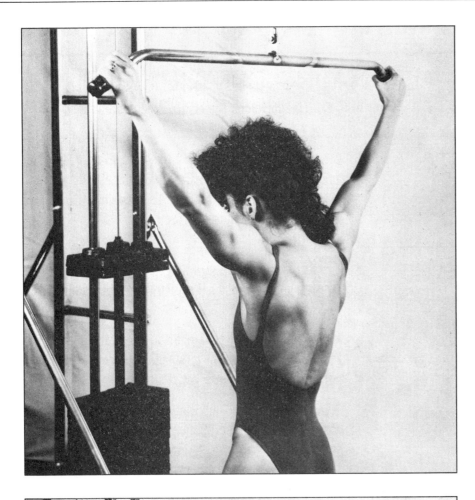

LAT MACHINE PULLDOWN
TO THE BACK (START)

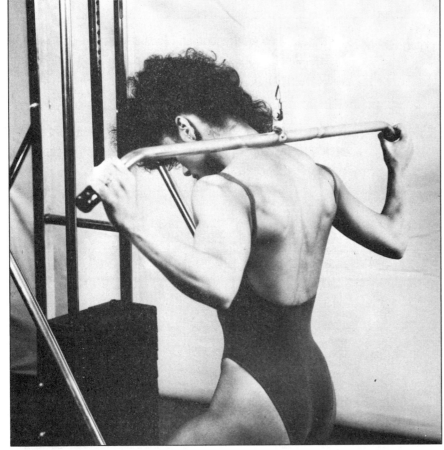

LAT MACHINE PULLDOWN
TO THE BACK (FINISH)

BICEPS ROUTINE

STANDING ALTERNATING DUMBBELL CURL

This exercise develops the entire biceps area.

DIRECTIONS	• Grasp one dumbbell in each hand, palms facing your sides and your arms straight down at your sides. (As you perform the exercise, be sure to keep your arms close to your sides at all times.)
MOVEMENT	• Turning your palm upward as you move, raise your right arm to shoulder height, keeping your elbow pinned to your waist.
	• As you are lowering your right arm to starting position, raise your left arm to shoulder height, turning your left palm upward as you go.
	• Repeat this right-left alternate movement until you have completed the correct number of repetitions for your set. (You will have raised and lowered the left arm 15 times, and you will have raised and lowered the right arm 15 times.)
SUGGESTIONS	Concentrate on contracting and flexing your biceps as you raise the dumbbell. Look at the muscle and watch it bulge as you contract it.
DON'TS	Do not sway from side to side, using your shoulders for momentum. Instead, stand still and use only your biceps to do the work. Concentrate. Work hard.

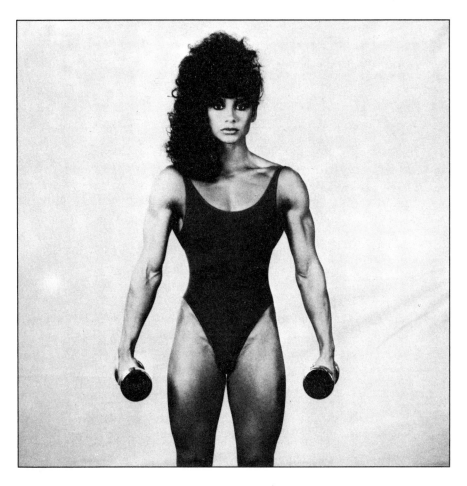

STANDING ALTERNATING
DUMBBELL CURL (START)

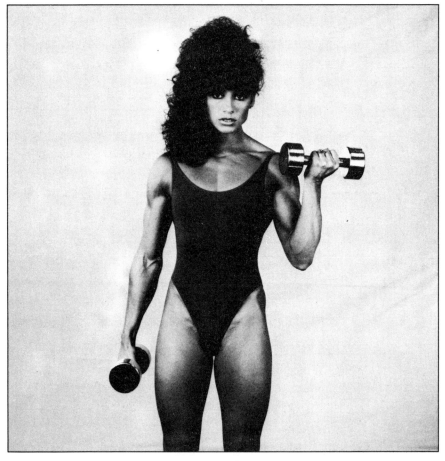

STANDING ALTERNATING
DUMBBELL CURL (FINISH)

CONCENTRATION CURL

This exercise develops the middle part (peak) of the biceps.

DIRECTIONS	• Take a dumbbell in your left hand and sit at a flat exercise bench with your feet about 2 feet apart. • Bend forward at the waist and place your left elbow, dumbbell held palm inward, on your left knee. • Let your arm hang straight down and allow the dumbbell to pull your arm toward the floor.
MOVEMENT	• Slowly move the dumbbell up until you have completely bent your elbow. (Be careful *not* to bend your wrist.) • Slowly lower the weight to starting position. (Be sure to remain bent at the waist. Do not sit up.) • Repeat the movement until you have performed the correct number of repetitions for your set, and then do the same for the other arm.
SUGGESTIONS	You will have to use a light weight until you get used to this exercise (probably as low as 5 or 8 pounds). Watch the biceps move up as you contract it and down as you expand it. Concentrate and flex (squeeze) as hard as you can on the upward movement.
DON'TS	Do not sit up. Lean down at all times. Never swing the weight up to give it momentum. Slowly raise it. Never let the weight drop down to starting position. Control it at all times. Concentrate.
INCLINE DUMBBELL CURL	Follow the exercise description on p. 90.
STANDING BARBELL CURL	Follow the exercise description on p. 92.
PULLEY CURL	Follow the exercise description on p. 96.

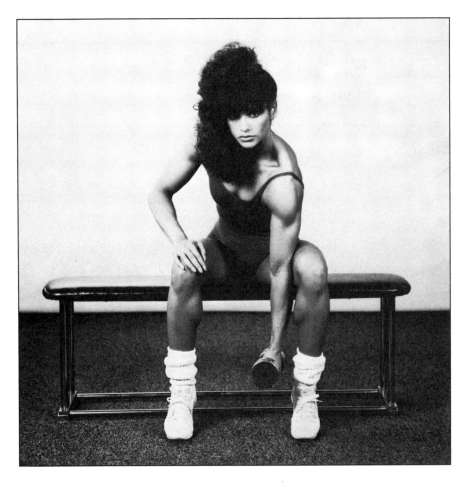

CONCENTRATION CURL (START)

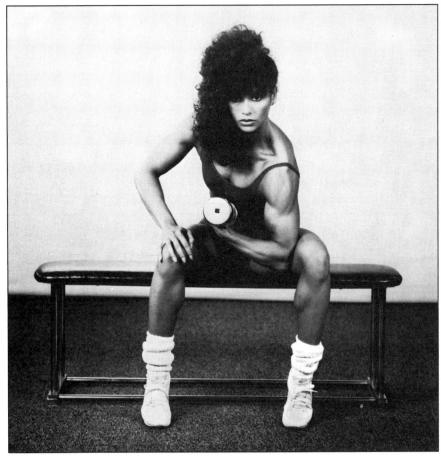

CONCENTRATION CURL (FINISH)

TRICEPS ROUTINE

PULLEY PUSHOUT—ONE ARM

This exercise develops the entire triceps area.

DIRECTIONS	• Place a triangular attachment to the upper pulley of the freestanding pulley machine. • Stand with your back to the pulley, holding the bar of the triangle in your right hand, palm forward. • Place your upper right arm close to your body, using your left hand to hold it there. (Cross your left hand over your body and grip your right arm near the biceps area.) Your right forearm should be pinned to your head near your ear. • Stand about 4 feet away from the pulley.
MOVEMENT	• Keeping your arm close to your body, slowly pull the bar out in front of you until you have fully extended your arm. • Keeping your head from dropping down (by looking straight ahead), slowly return to starting position and immediately repeat the movement until you have performed the correct number of repetitions for your set. • Repeat the set for your left arm.
SUGGESTIONS	Flex (squeeze together) your triceps as you perform the movement.
DON'TS	Do not let your elbow wander outward, away from your head. Be sure to feel the stress in your triceps area.
ONE-ARM DUMBBELL TRICEPS EXTENSION	Follow the exercise description on p. 102.
DIP BETWEEN BENCHES	Follow the exercise description on p. 100.
LYING TRICEPS EXTENSION	Follow the exercise description on p. 98.
PULLEY PUSHDOWN	Follow the exercise description on p. 104.

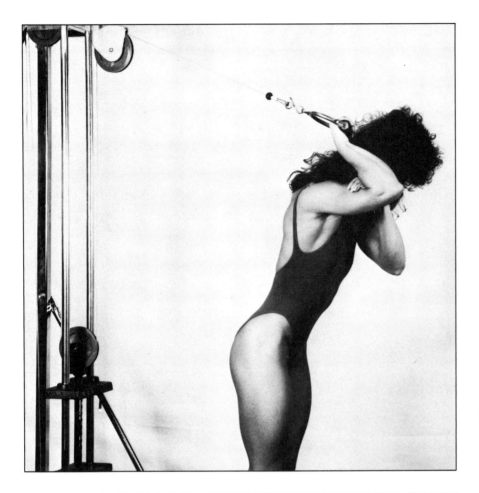

PULLEY PUSHOUT (START)

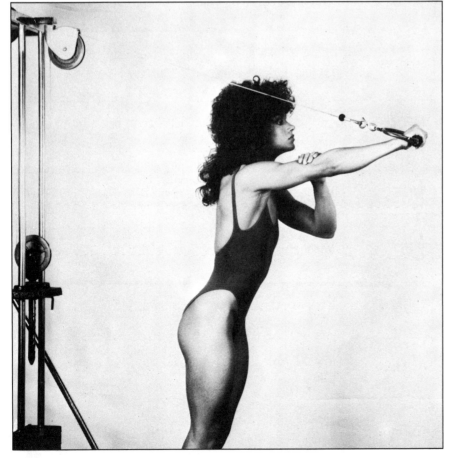

PULLEY PUSHOUT (FINISH)

LEG ROUTINE

CALF PRESS

This exercise develops the gastrocnemius (calf muscle) and is done on the leg press machine of the Universal Gym. (A substitute exercise can be done on any leg press machine.)

DIRECTIONS	• Sit in the seat of the machine and, with your feet in the shoeplates, adjust the machine so that you are six notches away from the closest position.
	• Place your feet on the shoeplates so that the balls of your feet center the lower rim of the shoeplates.
	• Extend your legs fully so that the pressure of the weight is felt fully by your feet.
MOVEMENT	• Thrust your toes forward slowly until your feet are fully extended, and then slowly allow your feet to return to starting position, bending your feet at the ankle as far back as possible.
	• Repeat this movement until you have performed the correct number of repetitions for your set.
SUGGESTIONS	Create a mental image of your calf muscle contracting and expanding as you perform the exercise.
DON'TS	Do not do this exercise without a good pair of gym shoes or sneakers.
LUNGE	Follow the exercise description on p. 106.
SQUAT	Follow the exercise description on p. 110.
LEG EXTENSION	Follow the exercise description on p. 112.
LEG CURL	Follow the exercise description on p. 114.

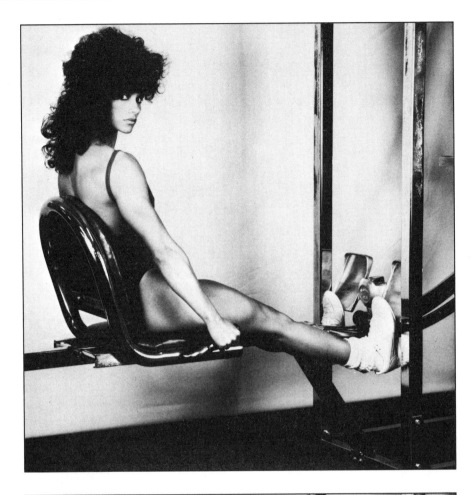

CALF PRESS (START)

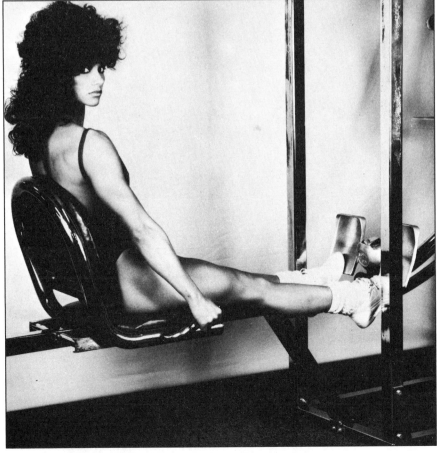

CALF PRESS (FINISH)

A B D O M I N A L   R O U T I N E

Abdominals require more work than any other body part. No matter what condition you are in, more time must be devoted to them. You'll exercise them every workout day.

Most abdominal exercises do not require the use of a weight, and those that do use a very light weight.

The first week you will do only 15 repetitions per set of each abdominal exercise. Beginning with the second week, add 5 repetitions per week until you have reached 25 repetitions per exercise. Remain at 25 repetitions for one month. Then you must again add 5 repetitions per week until you have reached 40 repetitions per set of each abdominal exercise. We recommend that you gradually increase to 50 repetitions per set.

It is extremely important for you bulky bodies to pay strict attention to the abdominal area because, as you well know, this is a favorite place for excess fat to deposit itself. It is only by hard and continual work that the abdominal area will give up its deposit of excess fat so that the muscles being formed can be revealed.

The reward of working your abdominals hard will be seen in the form of pretty, appealing muscles on the stomach instead of rolls of unsightly fat. It will be well worth it in the long run.

KNEE-UP

This exercise develops the lower abdominal muscles.

DIRECTIONS	• Lie on a flat exercise bench with your calves just about touching the end of the bench. • Place your hands under your buttocks and keep your legs extended straight out in front of you, raised off the bench.
MOVEMENT	• Slowly bend your knees, pulling them up until they almost touch your chest. • Immediately return to starting position (flexing your lower abdominals at all times) and repeat the movement until you have performed the correct number of repetitions for your set.
SUGGESTIONS	You may, after a few months, wish to try this exercise with a light weight (about 3 or 5 pounds) held between your feet. If you do, be careful to hold the weight securely at all times and remember to flex your lower abdominal muscles.
DON'TS	Do not jerk your legs up and let them fall down. Slowly raise your knees and lower them, concentrating on the formation of your lower abdominals. (Picture them taking shape. Remember the mental image in the mirror.)
STRAIGHT BENCH SIT-UP	Follow the exercise description on p. 120.
ROMAN CHAIR SIT-UP WITH A WEIGHT	Follow the exercise description on p. 122.
BENCH LEG RAISE WITH A WEIGHT	Follow the exercise description on p. 124, only do not use a weight. You may use a weight after 3 months if you wish.
SERRATUS PULL	Follow the exercise description on p. 126.
INCLINE BENCH LEG RAISE	Follow the exercise description on p. 118.
CRUNCH	Follow the exercise description on p. 144.

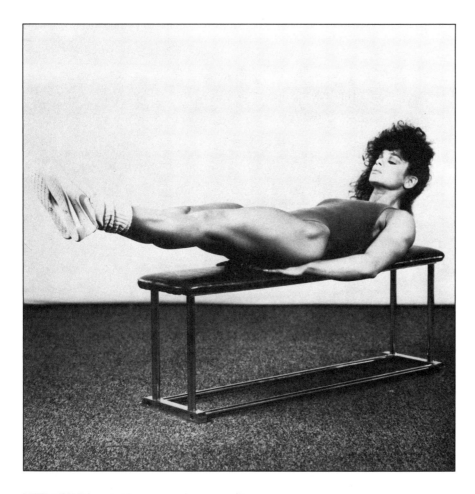

KNEE-UP (START)

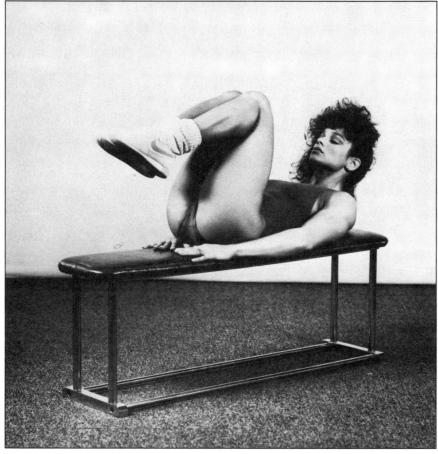

KNEE-UP (FINISH)

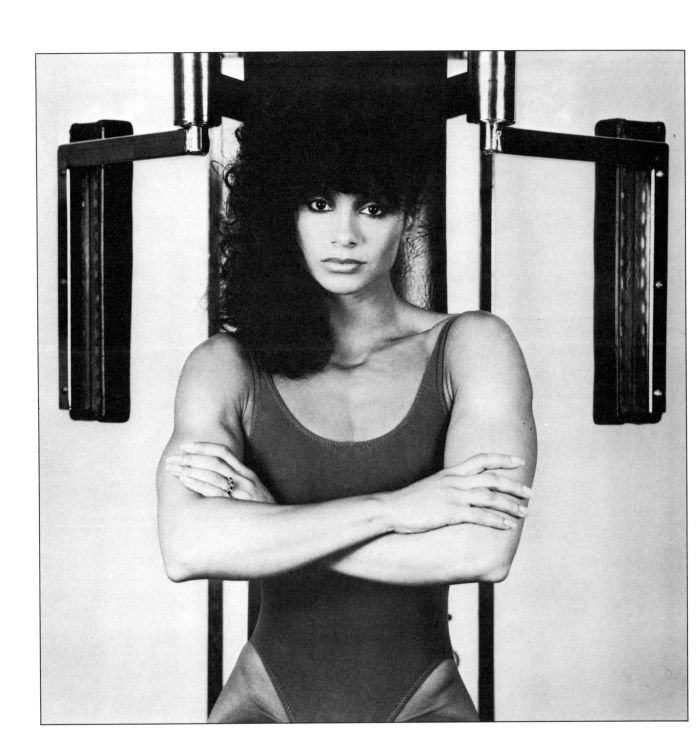

FINE-TUNING YOUR ROUTINE

Most women have a body area that has always been a problem for them. It can be a bulging stomach or large buttocks or lumpy hips or shapeless thighs or hanging triceps or sagging breasts. Nothing seems to help.

A hard body doesn't have any of these problems, and by following the workout for your body category you will see real improvements within three months. But if you want to speed things up, here are some ways to ensure visible results for your problem areas in less than half the time.

There are four principal trouble spots: abdomen, triceps, breasts, and hips-buttocks-thighs. You may say "I need help in all of those areas," but you must decide which one is of most importance and attack that one first.

WORKING THE TROUBLESOME AREA
FIRST IN YOUR ROUTINE

Regardless of what we suggest for your regular routine, you must start your workout with your "troublesome" area first. For example, if your abdomen is your problem area, begin your workout each workout day with that group of exercises. If the hip-buttock-thigh area is your problem, begin your workout, on the days you do legs, with legs. Our leg routine, you will remember, stresses muscles in the hips, buttocks, and thighs. When you begin each workout on your problem areas, you bring more concentration and fresher energy to the exercises for those areas.

MORE REPS

Another way to "bomb" your troublesome area is to add repetitions to the *last set* of each exercise for that area. Suppose, for example, that your troublesome area is your triceps, and you are an in-between body. The first exercise in your regular triceps routine is the lying triceps extension, and you would ordinarily complete 8–10 repetitions for your last set. Instead, you will squeeze out as many extra reps as possible on that last set, even if it means that you do not get a full movement. This form of "cheating" is beneficial, because it allows you to break a barrier. You may even feel a burning sensation in your triceps area as you force yourself to perform a few more reps. This means you're working the muscle to full capacity. Try to get between 5 and 10 extra reps for that last set. Squeeze out extra reps on the last set of each exercise for the body part you most want to improve.

MORE EXERCISES

You may have noticed that while there is some overlapping of exercises among the slim, in-between, and bulky body workouts, there are some exercises that are exclusive to each workout. Any of the exercises that are not part of your regular routine can be used as extra exercises. If you're feeling aggressive about launching a superintense attack on your hips and thighs, for example, find any exercise from the legs routine of the workouts you're *not* engaged in. Add it to your regular workout. In other words, you'll have one more exercise for your legs routine. So whether your problem is hips-thighs-buttocks, triceps, abdominals, or breasts, you can find more exercises in either of the two workouts you're not using.

HOW MUCH IS TOO MUCH?

It must be reiterated that the basic slim, in-between, and bulky body workouts are complete programs for shaping your body into a hard body of perfect proportions. But if you really want to see a faster transformation, any of these fine-tuning techniques can be incorporated into your routine. The easiest is rearranging the sequence of your exercises to start your routine by working your trouble spot. Then move on to squeezing out a few more reps at the end of the last set of one or two exercises. Increase the number of extra reps gradually.

Only after you've worked up to 10 extra reps on two exercises should you consider adding another exercise to your routine. Since you always complete 3 sets of an exercise, adding 1 to your routine is a substantial commitment. Adding more than 2 is too much!

Because the hips-buttocks-thighs are so stubborn, we have developed a daily floor exercise routine that can be done at home. This routine should be performed at a convenient time, usually in the morning or just before bedtime. The whole routine takes 10–15 minutes. It is not strenuous, yet it hits away at lumpy hips, loose buttocks, and shapeless thighs. You may choose to do this routine in addition to the above suggestions, or simply to follow your regular leg routine for hips, buttocks, and thighs and add this daily floor routine.

The focus of each exercise is described. You may select as many as you want. Remember to work your way gradually into a full program.

Do 3 sets of each exercise. Start out with 10 repetitions for each set. Add 1 repetition to a set until you are doing 15 repetitions per set. This should take no longer than 3 weeks. If you feel ambitious, you may go as high as 25 repetitions per set, but 15 repetitions will achieve excellent results.

SIDE LEG RAISE

This exercise tightens the back thighs and the buttocks.

DIRECTIONS	• Lie on the floor on your left side, your body completely extended, your right hip tilted forward approximately 45 degrees. • Place your left hand behind your neck, and your left elbow on the floor for support. Place your right palm on the floor in front of your breast area for support. Keep toes pointed away from you. • Place your right foot behind the left foot, the arch of the right foot touching the heel of your left foot.
MOVEMENT	• With knees locked, lifting from the tightened buttocks and flexed (squeezed together) thigh, raise your right leg as high as possible and quickly return to starting position. • Repeat this movement until you have completed the correct number of repetitions for your set. • Repeat the movement for the other side of your body.
SUGGESTIONS	This exercise is easy enough so that you can quickly advance to at least 25 repetitions. Many women go as high as 50 repetitions. Be sure to keep your buttock and thigh flexed (squeezed together) at all times during the movement. It may be more comfortable to lie flat on your extended arm instead of placing it behind your neck, especially if you have back problems.
DON'TS	Do not bend your knee while performing the movement. Do not relax your thigh or buttocks. Keep them flexed and perform the movement in a strict manner.

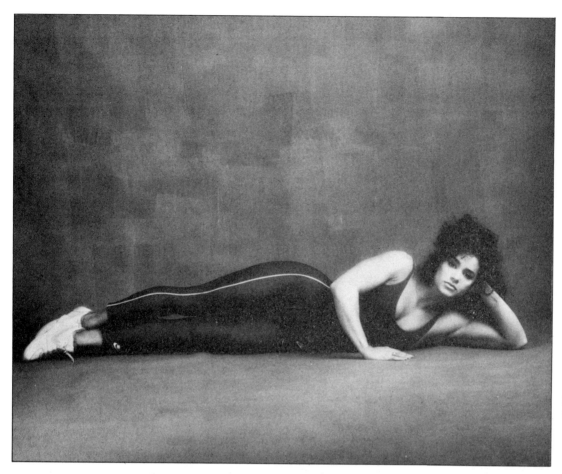

SIDE LEG RAISE
(START)

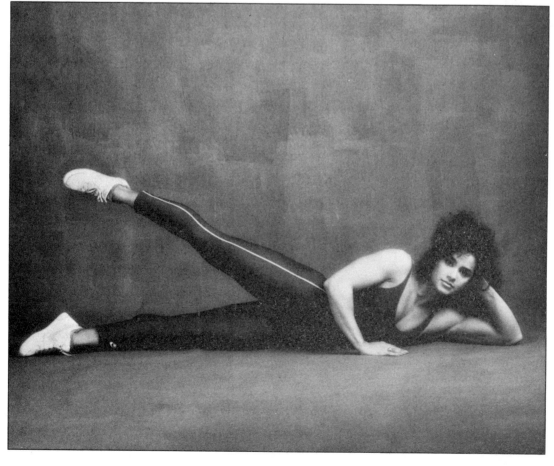

SIDE LEG RAISE
(FINISH)

SIDE LEG LIFT

This exercise helps eliminate excess bulges from the hip area and reduce excess fat from the inner thigh.

DIRECTIONS

- Place your body in an all-fours position, resting on your knees, with your arms fully extended, elbows locked.

- Extend your right leg straight out to your side at a 45-degree angle to your body, and flex your foot toward your body.

MOVEMENT

- With knee locked, raise your extended right leg 4–8 inches off the floor (as high as possible) and quickly lower it to starting position.

- Without resting your foot on the floor, quickly repeat the movement until you have performed the correct number of repetitions for your set.

- Repeat the movement for your left leg.

SUGGESTIONS

This is a difficult movement and you may find it necessary to do only 10 repetitions per set for the first week.

DON'TS

Do not tilt your hip toward the nonworking leg to make the movement easier. Keep your hips parallel to the floor at all times. Do not bend your knee, but keep it locked throughout the movement.

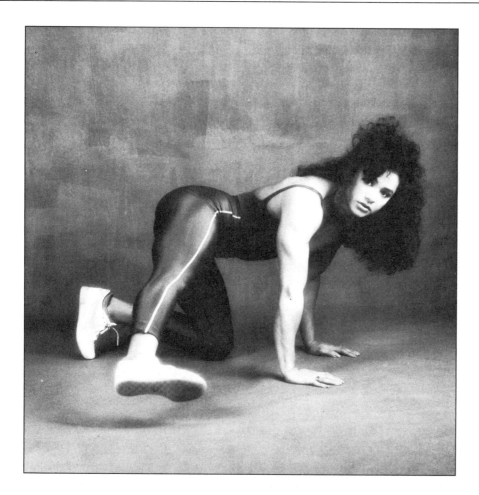

SIDE LEG LIFT (START)

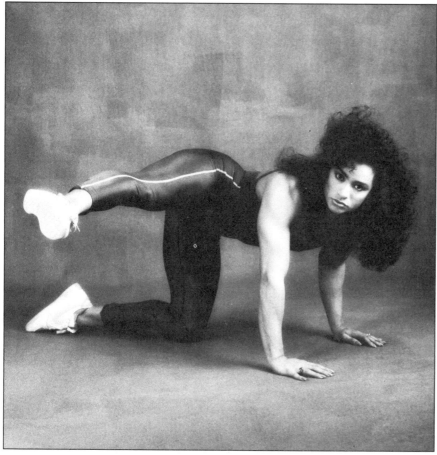

SIDE LEG LIFT (FINISH)

FIRE HYDRANT

This exercise helps tighten the buttocks and the inner and outer thigh area.

DIRECTIONS

- Place your body in an all-fours position, resting on your knees, arms fully extended and elbows locked.

- Be sure that your back is parallel to the floor (not arched or swayed downward).

- Lift your right hip 2 inches. Your knee will also be 2 inches off the floor. The knee is not to touch the floor until the required number of repetitions for that leg are performed.

MOVEMENT

- The movement of this exercise takes place in four steps:
  1. Extend right thigh out (keeping knee-to-ankle bent as it was in the kneeling position).
  2. In that position, extend knee-to-ankle straight out so that your entire leg is extended out to your side at a 90-degree angle.
  3. Bend knee-to-ankle back to Step 1 position.
  4. Return knee to floor. (You are now back in the all-fours starting position.)

- Repeat this four-step movement until you have completed the correct number of repetitions for your set.

- Repeat the movement for your left leg.

SUGGESTIONS

Remember to flex (tighten) your thigh and buttock areas while performing the movement.

DON'TS

Do not rest your knee on the floor between repetitions. Keep your knee about two inches off the floor (when returning to starting position).

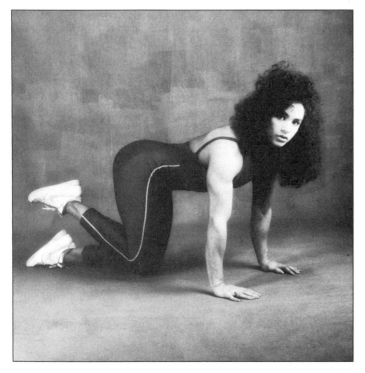

FIRE HYDRANT (START)

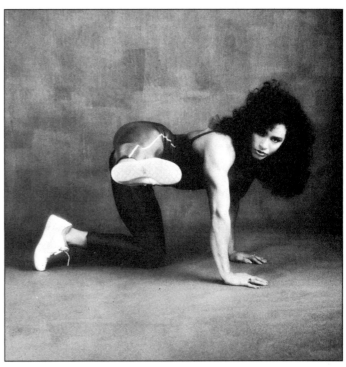

FIRE HYDRANT (STEP 2)

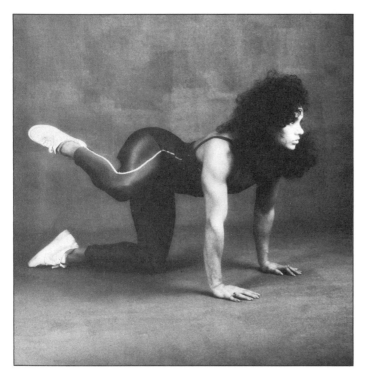

FIRE HYDRANT (STEP 1)

BACK LEG KICK

This exercise helps to tighten the buttocks and the back thigh areas.

DIRECTIONS	• Place your body in an all-fours position, resting on your knees, arms fully extended, elbows locked.
	• Extend your right leg straight out behind you, and flex your foot toward you.
	• Keep your back as parallel to the floor as possible throughout the movement.
MOVEMENT	• Lifting from the tightened buttocks, raise your right leg (knee locked) as high as possible and quickly lower it to starting position. Immediately repeat the movement, never letting your foot touch the floor between the repetitions, until you have completed the correct number of repetitions for your set.
	• Repeat the movement for your left leg.
SUGGESTIONS	Be sure to keep your hips and buttocks flexed (squeezed together), your knee locked and your elbows locked. Remember to keep your hips parallel to the floor.
DON'TS	Do not move your upper body during the exercise. Keep your back from swaying downward or arching upward. Do not lose the parallel-to-the-floor position of your back while performing the kicking motion.

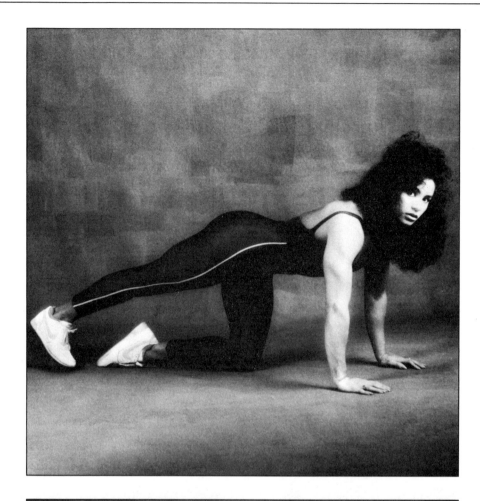

BACK LEG KICK (START)

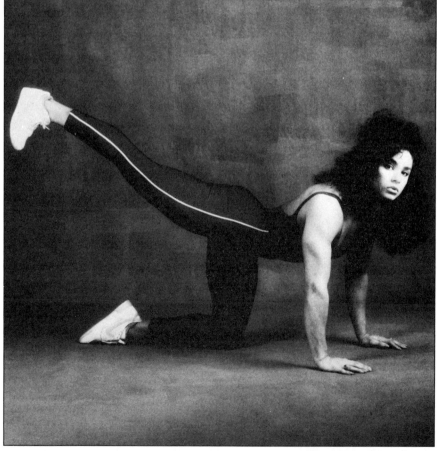

BACK LEG KICK (FINISH)

SCISSORS

This exercise helps to tighten the outer thigh and lower hips area, the inner thigh area, and the lower abdominals.

DIRECTIONS	• Lie flat on your back, resting your head on the floor.
	• Place your palms flat on the floor under your buttocks and raise your legs, knees locked, almost perpendicular to the floor.
	• Turn your knees outward and point your toes out at a 45-degree angle. There should be a one-inch space between your heels.

| MOVEMENT | • Move both legs out as far as possible, keeping the knees locked and your inner and outer thighs flexed. |
| | • Return to starting position, but do not cross your legs over each other. Immediately repeat the movement. |

| SUGGESTIONS | This is a rather easy movement, so you may find that you can start out with 25 repetitions and work your way up to 50 repetitions per set. |

| DON'TS | Do not jerk your legs out abruptly. Rather, with flexed thighs (inner and outer) move rapidly out as far as possible and then back in to starting position. Jerking can cause muscle pulls. Control the movement and concentrate at all times. |

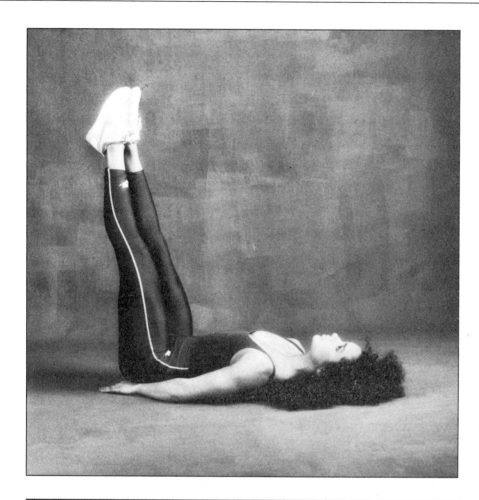

SCISSORS (START)

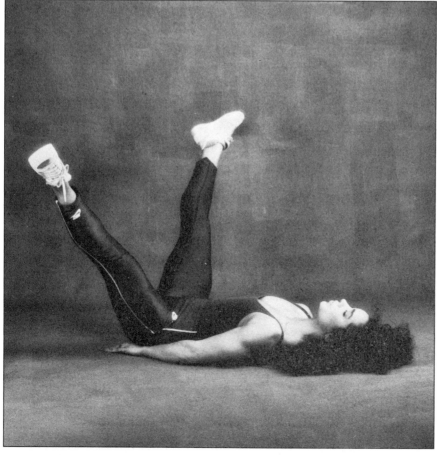

SCISSORS (FINISH)

REVIEW OF THE FINE-TUNING ATTACK

ABDOMINAL AREA	1. Work the abdominals first. 2. Add extra repetitions to the last set of each exercise. 3. Add one or two exercises.
TRICEPS	1. Work the triceps first. 2. Add extra repetitions to the last set of each exercise. 3. Add one or two exercises.
BREASTS	1. Work the chest first. 2. Add extra repetitions to the last set of each exercise. 3. Add one or two exercises.
HIPS, BUTTOCKS, THIGHS	1. Work the legs first. (This area includes hips, buttocks, and thighs.) 2. Add extra repetitions to the last set of each exercise. 3. Add one or two exercises. 4. Do the floor exercises daily.
SUMMARY	You may do any or all of the above, but we suggest that you do them in the order given (except for the floor exercises, which can be added at any time).

RESULTS

Combining these "bombing" techniques with your workout will get you results quickly. After about three months you should see a real difference in the troublesome area. You may choose to continue bombing the area or you may drop the extra work. Your regular routine will hold you once you've beaten the troublesome area into shape.

CONCENTRATION AND VISUALIZATION

Don't forget to concentrate while doing each repetition of each set of your exercises. Your goal is to remove the problem, whether it be loose skin, bulges, or bunched-up fat, and to replace that problem with a perfectly formed body part. For this reason you must flex (squeeze, tighten) the particular muscle you are working. Do not neglect to picture that muscle expanding and contracting as you work it. Look at the muscle in the mirror whenever possible as it contracts and expands during the exercise. Or else have a mental picture of the muscle growing and taking shape. Mentally tell the muscle what form it should take. Don't forget to stand in front of the mirror at least once a week, in a bikini or in the nude, and resculpt your muscles mentally into your perfect hard body.

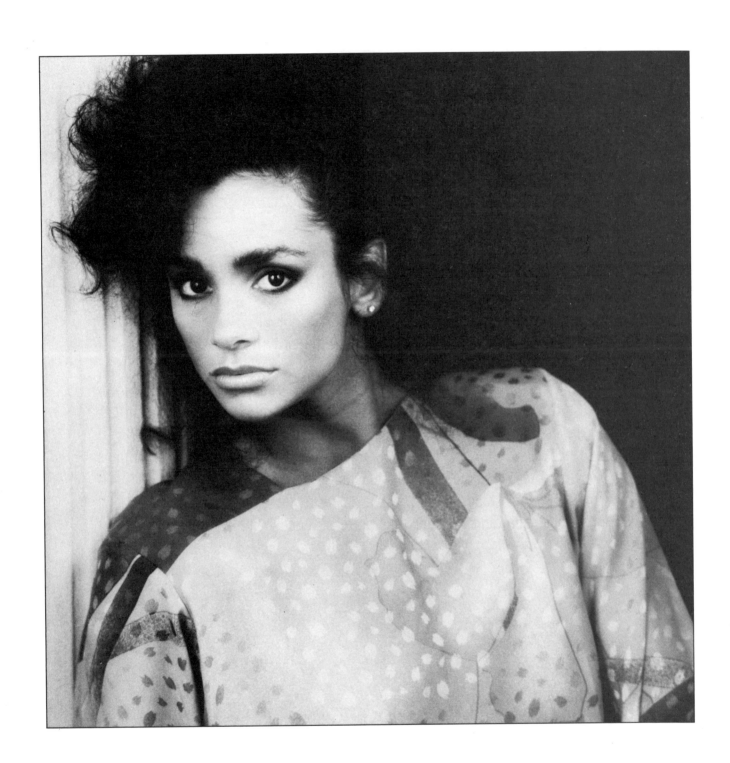

THE HARD BODIES DIET

It is possible to eat delicious, nutritious food and not get fat. There is no reason ever to be hungry when correct eating habits are established. Forget the years of struggle and learn to enjoy food again.

Before describing the weight loss, weight gain, and weight maintenance diets, we would like to explain some food basics. Food is measured in calories. A calorie is the amount of chemical *energy* that can be released as heat when food is metabolized. It follows, then, that food which is high in calories is also high in energy value. Fats, for example, yield approximately nine calories per gram, while carbohydrates and protein yield only four calories per gram.

To make the picture simple, it takes approximately 3,500 calories to add one pound of fat to your body. So if you want to gain one pound, you must eat 3,500 calories more than usual. This may be accomplished in three days, four days, a week, however long it takes to consume the extra 3,500 calories. The system, of course, works in reverse. To lose one pound, you must eat 3,500 fewer calories than usual, and this too can be accomplished in a few days, a week, or longer, depending upon how much food you are willing to give up.

Weight is a mystery to some women. We've become slaves to the scale, that instrument that can only weigh mass with no distinction between muscle and fat. The inadequacy of the scale becomes clear when we realize that muscle weighs at least twice as much as fat. For example, a piece of fat will weigh much less than a piece of red meat the same size. When a woman's body consists of lots of fat, say 35 percent, she can be of the same height and weight as another whose body contains only 15 percent fat. The woman with the higher fat content will be larger because fat displaces more volume.

After spending time with the Hard Bodies workout, you will shed body fat and replace it with muscle. You'll look much slimmer as the fat disappears, but since you are also adding muscle—which weighs more and yet takes up less space—the scale will usually not show a major weight loss.

The principles to remember at all times are:

MUSCLE WEIGHS MORE THAN FAT.

A POUND OF MUSCLE TAKES UP LESS ROOM THAN A POUND OF FAT.

MUSCLE IS SHAPELY AND FAT IS SHAPELESS.

So don't become discouraged if the scales aren't dipping.

Foods are made up of three basic elements: carbohydrates, proteins, and fats. The Hard Bodies diet requires a basic understanding of their roles in good nutrition.

FATS

In spite of its bad reputation, fat is an absolute necessity for good nutrition and health. Without fats vitamins A, D, E, and K would not be metabolized. Without fat vitamin D would not be absorbed by the body. Calcium would be unavailable to the tissues and bones and teeth.

Fat also serves as a cushion for our internal organs. It forms a layer around them, protecting them from injury which would otherwise occur at the slightest jogging movement. The thin layer of fat under the skin protects us from the cold by retaining body heat.

It is highly unlikely that anyone reading this book has a problem of too little body fat. In fact, the American diet is so high in fat that most people consume 45 percent of their calories in fat. A healthier level of calories in fat is 15–20 percent.

As mentioned, one gram of fat produces 9 calories. Look at the fat content of these favorite foods:

QUANTITY	FOOD	GRAMS OF FAT
1	thick shake	16
1	medium order french fries	20
1 slice	pie	20
1 tbs	peanut butter	7.5
1 tbs	butter	12
1 oz	cream cheese	9
1 tbs	French dressing	5
1 tbs	Italian dressing	9
3	Oreo cookies	7

Even the most unlikely foods contain fat. Eating vegetables, fruits, and lean meats will provide the average person with more than enough fat for the daily requirement (which will be discussed later). Even these "thin" foods contain some fat:

AMOUNT	FOOD	GRAMS OF FAT
8-oz can	pineapple, in own juice	.3
1	apple	1
1 cup	carrots	1
1 lb	fresh spinach	1.6
1 cup	strawberries	1
4 oz	white-meat chicken, broiled without skin	5

Your total diet should consist of no more than about 15 percent fat. If you are allowing yourself, say, 2,000 calories a day, this means you are allowed only 300 calories of fat, or 33.3 grams.

Think of what a medium order of fries, a thick shake, and a salad with Italian dressing would do to your fat intake. That would be 567 calories (63 grams) of fat, almost double your allowed intake (assuming you had 3 tbs of salad dressing) —all in one meal.

We suggest that you purchase a copy of *The Nutrition Almanac* or *The at a Glance Nutrition Counter* (listed in the bibliography) to help you keep track of your fat intake.

CARBOHYDRATES

Carbohydrates are the body's main source of energy. They also help metabolize protein and fat. It is said that fats burn with the fuel of carbohydrates. Without carbohydrates, fats could not be broken down in the liver, and digestive problems would occur.

There are basically three kinds of carbohydrates: simple carbohydrates found in fruits, complex carbohydrates found in vegetables, grains, and seeds, and processed carbohydrates found in sugars, honeys, syrups, candy, cake and other sweets.

SIMPLE CARBOHYDRATES

Simple carbohydrates are found in fruits and provide immediate energy because they are quickly metabolized and go straight into the bloodstream.

COMPLEX CARBOHYDRATES

Vegetables, grains, and whole grains contain complex carbohydrates. Such carbohydrates provide gradually released energy because they require prolonged enzymatic action to be broken down into simple sugars for digestion. The value of complex carbohydrates over simple carbohydrates is their ability to provide a continual energy supply with their gradual release.

Both simple and complex carbohydrates are converted into glucose, which is used by the brain, the nervous system, and muscles. Some of it is stored, for reserved energy, in the muscles and liver as glycogen. Excess glucose is stored in the body as fat. Hence, it is important not to eat excess carbohydrates when the goal is weight loss. When caloric intake is reduced, the body reconverts the fat into glucose to be used as fuel for energy. It is "burned up," and excess body fat is reduced—along with weight.

PROCESSED CARBOHYDRATES

The processed carbohydrates, which are found in candy, cake, ice cream, and other sweets, provide you with a quick shot of immediate energy. The problem is, they cause a sudden rise in the blood sugar level. The energy lasts for a short time, perhaps fifteen minutes, while the blood sugar level is high. Suddenly, however, the blood sugar drops. That high energy is replaced by a feeling of weakness and fatigue. To stay "up" you are drawn to another "fix" of processed sugar. The result is overeating of processed sugars—which are very high in calories—and weight gain. In short, stay away from processed sugars.

IDEAL SIMPLE AND COMPLEX CARBOHYDRATES

SIMPLE CARBOHYDRATES	COMPLEX CARBOHYDRATES
cantaloupe	potato
honeydew	mushroom
grapefruit	tomato
peach	carrot
pineapple	peas
apple	lettuce
strawberry	cucumber
plum	squash
pear	green pepper
cherry	cauliflower
	rice, white (unpolished)
	rice, brown
	whole grain bread

Carbohydrates are vital for good health. They contribute to mental and physical stamina. We urge our readers to avoid the low-carbohydrate, high-protein diets that periodically become popular. Such diets leave you fatigued and unhealthy. In that condition it is too easy to reach for a quick hit of energy from a processed carbohydrate (cake, cookies, candy). You'll only end up gaining body fat and weight.

PROTEIN

Protein is the main component of body tissue, muscle in particular. Without it, muscles, blood, skin, hair, nails, and the organs such as the heart and brain could not exist and thrive. Protein also controls growth, sexual development, and metabolism. It is the main building material of the body.

We recommend that you consume three quarters of a gram of protein daily per pound of body weight. For example, if you weigh 120 pounds, you should take in 90 grams of protein or 360 calories in protein daily.

The protein in the muscles consists of 22 components, or "building blocks," called amino acids. The body can make 14 of these amino acids from any food, but the other 8 can be supplied only by certain protein-providing foods. These foods are called "complete protein" foods.

The foods containing the 8 essential amino acids are also the best sources of protein:

milk and milk products
eggs
fish
poultry
red meat

Sources of protein that contain some but not all of the 8 essential amino acids:
corn
rice
beans
vegetables
fruits

It may be surprising to discover that vegetables and fruits do indeed contain protein, but the amount is minute and the essential amino acids are not all present. There are ways of combining incomplete proteins such as rice and beans to form complete protein, but for perfected muscular development we suggest the intake of the complete proteins.

SODIUM

Before we discuss the ideal ratio of protein to fat and carbohydrates in your diet, it is important to understand the function of sodium.

Sodium is a mineral and is found in the body fluids and the bones. It assists digestion and is the main source of fluid regulation within the body. Other functions of sodium are the prevention of deposits from minerals in the bloodstream, the maintenance of blood chemistry balance, and purification of the body from poisonous carbon dioxide. Sodium also plays a part in muscle contraction and expansion and nerve stimulation. Without sodium the human body would dysfunction.

Lack of sodium is not a problem in the modern world. There is sodium (in the form of sodium chloride, or salt) in virtually every food, unprocessed, in its natural state. Tap water contains sodium. Most people ingest 3 to 7 grams of sodium a day, 3 to 5 times the ideal amount.

Hard bodies don't need excess sodium. Never use table salt. Stay away from high-sodium foods. Soon your taste buds will tell you when a food is high in sodium. In the meantime consult *The Nutrition Almanac* and look up the sodium contents of foods you eat.

The list of high sodium foods is endless, but here are some main offenders:

AMOUNT	FOOD	MILLIGRAMS OF SODIUM
1 tsp	table salt	2,000
1 cup	chow mein	1,675
1 cup	cottage cheese	900
1	pickle	930
1 cup	soup, canned (average)	1,000
1 cup	tomato juice	875

By means of contrast, here are some low-sodium foods:

QUANTITY	FOOD	MILLIGRAMS OF SODIUM
1 ear	corn on the cob	1
1	baked potato	5
4 oz	white-meat chicken, broiled without skin	87
1	large apple	2
½	cantaloupe	24
1	large orange	1
1	large pear	0

Limit your sodium intake to foods that naturally contain sodium; avoid canned foods completely. Fresh foods are always best, but if time and convenience demand the intake of prepared foods, use frozen rather than canned. There are 450 milligrams of sodium in a cup of *canned* peas and carrots but only 50 in a cup of *frozen* peas and carrots.

THE BALANCED DIET

The healthy, balanced diet consists of the following:

15 percent fat
67 percent carbohydrate
18 percent protein

Translated into calories, using the example of a 120-pound woman who is on a 2,000-calorie maintenance diet, the balanced diet looks like this:

  300 calories in fat
1,340 calories in carbohydrate
  360 calories in protein

A day's meal could look like this:

BREAKFAST
2–poached eggs
2 slices whole wheat toast
1 cup coffee with skim milk
1 glass orange juice (8 oz)

SNACK
1 bran muffin

LUNCH
6 oz cottage cheese (low-fat, low-sodium)
1 slice whole wheat bread
lettuce and tomato salad with vinegar
1 apple
1 cup skim milk

SNACK
1 peach

DINNER
4 oz white-meat chicken breast, skinned
1 cup peas
1 cup carrots
1 cup high-protein spaghetti
½ cup spaghetti sauce (Ragú Homestyle)
½ grapefruit

The above menu measures approximately as follows:
  300 calories in fat (75 grams fat)
1,340 calories in carbohydrate (335 grams carbohydrate)
  360 calories in protein (90 grams protein)

The balanced diet is the only way to avoid bingeing and the need for quick hits of energy from processed sugars. There is no need to become fanatical about the proportions of fat, protein, and carbohydrates. Allow yourself five percent leeway in any category; it won't make a big difference.

Try to spread out the 90 grams of protein over several meals, because it is impossible for the body to digest more than 30 grams at one time.

WEIGHT LOSS DIET

To lose weight, it is necessary to reduce the caloric intake over a period of time by 3,500 calories for each pound of weight loss. The most intelligent way to go about this reduction is *gradually*.

Reduce your caloric intake, from what it is now, by 100 calories a day until you are consuming 1,500 calories a day. This may take a week to ten days. Of course, you will need to calculate how much you are eating now by looking up the caloric values of the foods you consume in *The Nutrition Almanac* or another calorie counter.

It is not possible to lose more than two or two and a half pounds of body fat per week. If a woman loses more than two pounds a week, she is losing lean tissue and water. Such a loss is never good. This occurs when you try to diet too quickly and literally starve your body with less than 900 calories per day. The inevitable result is failure and an urge to binge.

Weight loss can also be achieved by burning up 3,500 calories for every pound of fat lost—through extra work or exercise. Everything we do requires the use of energy. Even sleeping uses up 60 calories an hour, and sitting in a chair reading burns up 70 calories an hour. Desk work takes 130 calories an hour. But what a slow way to lose weight. Consider these activities:

ACTIVITY	CALORIE LOSS PER HOUR
running	800
swimming	600

Hard Bodies workout	700
skiing	700
tennis	350

If you add to your daily routine an exercise that burns up 500 calories, you will lose one pound of body fat per week. If you give up 500 calories of food, you will lose another pound per week. There you have a two-pound weight loss each week.

Eat low-fat, low-sodium, sugarless foods. Select from fresh and frozen vegetables. Arrange your plate to have a variety of colors. Carrots, broccoli, and corn make a pretty platter. Satisfy your sweet tooth legitimately with fresh fruits. If grapefruits are not sweet enough, try pineapples. Cherries may be a little higher in calories than cantaloupe, but still a lot lower than ice cream or candy. Peaches, pears, apples, plums, nectarines, and even grapes are fair game. Grapes are a bit high, but again, not compared to cake or doughnuts.

How fast you lose weight will depend upon many factors. To review: weight loss depends upon a caloric deficiency of 3,500 calories per pound of body fat lost. However, when working with weights, the body is losing fat and gaining muscle at the same time. Since muscle weighs more than fat, the scale may not show a drop as fast as you are actually losing fat. Your body, however, will show an obvious difference. Your size will be reduced. You'll look thinner, more athletically proportioned.

Here are some high-quality low-calorie foods:

MEATS
White-meat chicken, skin removed   lean veal cutlet
White-meat turkey, skin removed

FISH

| flounder | cod |
| sole | tuna in water |

CARBOHYDRATES, SIMPLE

apple	cantaloupe	raspberries	pineapple
orange	peach	blackberries	plum
grapefruit	strawberry	cranberries	pomegranate
nectarine	papaya	mango	

CARBOHYDRATES, COMPLEX

lettuce	artichoke
tomato	asparagus
radishes	zucchini
red or green pepper	turnip
spinach	cucumber
carrots	potato
peas	

CARBOHYDRATES, RICE AND GRAINS

rice, white (unpolished)	bran
rice, brown	oatmeal
spaghetti (protein)	shredded wheat
whole wheat bread	puffed rice
protein bread	puffed wheat

CONDIMENTS

all spices except salt
lemon
vinegar, all flavors
white wine used in cooking

The weight loss dieters can also eat any of the foods on the weight gain list, as long as they calculate the calories into their daily allowance of 1,500 calories.

WEIGHT GAIN DIET

To gain weight, your daily caloric intake must increase by 500 calories a day. But you will be working out at the same time and spending more energy than before. However, since you will be losing fat and gaining muscle, which is heavier than fat, an increase of 500 calories a day—even with the additional calories burned—should show up on a scale as about a pound of weight gain a week.

You are less concerned with what the scale says than with how you look in the mirror. The goal is to shape perfect proportions, not to reach a certain weight.

The only way to increase the daily caloric intake is gradually. We suggest that you increase your daily caloric intake (after you have calculated your approximate present daily caloric intake) by 100 calories a day until you have increased it by 500 calories.

Gaining weight, in your case, does not mean gaining "fat" weight. Since you're on the Hard Bodies program, your weight gain will be strictly muscle. For this reason, it is most important that you remember to abide by the guidelines for a balanced diet: 15 percent fat, 67 percent carbohydrate, and 18 percent protein. Don't work against your workout with shakes and fries and sweets.

Here are some high-quality high-caloried foods:

MEAT

lean ground round	lamb
sirloin	dark-meat chicken
round roast	dark-meat turkey
liver	

FISH

bluefish
salmon
mackerel

CARBOHYDRATES, SIMPLE

avocado	cherries
dates	plantain
honeydew	watermelon
pears	

CARBOHYDRATES, COMPLEX

corn on the cob	corn muffins
collard greens	whole wheat bagels
sweet potato	beets
bran muffins	

The weight gain diet will of course include all the foods listed on the weight loss diet, because those foods also provide maximum nutrition. The foods listed above, however, are higher in calories than those listed on the weight loss diet, and they provide the highest possible nutritional value.

MAINTENANCE DIET

Those of you who are already within the limits of your ideal weight will want to follow the maintenance diet. Here are guidelines on how many calories you can consume to hold that weight. Of course, the caloric allowance cannot be foolproof, and you will have to experiment. People have different metabolisms and burn energy at different rates.

YOUR WEIGHT	CALORIES ALLOWED
100 pounds	1,725
110 pounds	1,850
120 pounds	1,975
130 pounds	2,100
140 pounds	2,225
150 pounds	2,350

Depending upon your metabolism, the caloric allowance can vary by 50 calories in either direction.

The ideal amount of body fat on a woman should be approximately 20 percent. Many women who are at their ideal weight carry as much as 35 percent body fat. These are the women who look great in clothing but who hate to be seen in a bathing suit. They have a thin layer of fat on their thighs, hips, stomach, arms, and it is spongy and unpleasant to the touch.

Your goal on the maintenance diet is to bring your body gradually down to about 20 percent body fat. The only way to do this is to adhere to the balanced diet of 15 percent fat, 67 percent carbohydrate and 18 percent protein; to monitor your total calorie intake; and to train according to the in-between body routine. What you eat makes a difference. Your daily caloric intake, if consumed in thick shakes and hamburgers (high-fat foods), produce a fat body, not a hard body.

You may eat all the foods listed for the weight loss and the weight gain diets, as well as other foods you desire (be sure to look them up in *The Nutrition Almanac* or another food-value guide). Remember, always stay within your daily caloric allowance and the food-group percentage balance.

MUSCLE BURNS MORE THAN FAT

Muscle actually metabolizes food more quickly than does fat. If a woman has a high percentage of body fat, her metabolism is sluggish and she cannot eat as much as a person of the same weight and height without negative consequences. Put simply, fat burns calories slowly and inefficiently. The calories from a slice of bread are burned up more quickly by a woman with 20 percent body fat than by a woman with 30 percent body fat—if both are engaged in the same physical activity.

The goal of the Hard Bodies diet, then, is to achieve a lowered body fat percentage so your metabolism will speed up a bit and you can eat more calories without consequence and without having to pay for them with extra aerobics.

WHEN TO EAT

Eating less than an hour before a workout can negatively affect your performance. When first eaten, food is being "burned" or digested in your system. The circulatory system is busy working on the food and cannot generate the full amount of energy required for the workout. It is best to work out first and then eat. If you must eat before, it is best to wait two hours before going to the gym (although some women find they can eat a light meal and work out one hour later).

BIBLIOGRAPHY

Brody, Jane. *Jane Brody's The New York Times Guide to Personal Health.* New York: Avon Books, 1982.

Friedberg, Ardy. *Reach for It.* New York: Simon & Schuster, 1983.

Haas, Dr. Robert. *Eat to Win.* New York: Rawson Associates, 1983.

Hausman, Patricia. *The at a Glance Nutrition Counter.* New York: Ballantine Books, 1984.

Kirshbaum, John D. *The Nutrition Almanac.* New York: McGraw-Hill, 1979.

Reynolds, Bill, and Joyce Vedral. *Supercut: The Bodybuilder's Diet.* Chicago: Contemporary Books, 1985.

Weider, Joe, ed., *Bodybuilding and Conditioning for Women.* Chicago, Contemporary Books, 1983.

Weider, Joe, ed., *Nutrition and Training for Women Bodybuilders.* Chicago: Contemporary Books, 1984.

MAGAZINES

Flex, 2100 Erwin Street, Woodland Hills, CA 91367

Muscle and Fitness, 2100 Erwin Street, Woodland Hills, CA 91367

Shape, 2100 Erwin Street, Woodland Hills, CA 91367